Acute Care Surgery

Editor

GEORGE C. VELMAHOS

SURGICAL CLINICS
OF NORTH AMERICA

www.surgical.theclinics.com

Consulting Editor
RONALD F. MARTIN

February 2014 • Volume 94 • Number 1

ELSEVIER

1600 John F. Kennedy Boulevard • Suite 1800 • Philadelphia, Pennsylvania, 19103-2899

http://www.surgical.theclinics.com

SURGICAL CLINICS OF NORTH AMERICA Volume 94, Number 1
February 2014 ISSN 0039-6109, ISBN-13: 978-0-323-26682-6

Editor: John Vassallo, j.vassallo@elsevier.com

Developmental Editor: Yonah Korngold

Surgical Clinics of North America (ISSN 0039-6109) is published bimonthly by Elsevier Inc., 360 Park Avenue South, New York, NY 10010-1710. Months of publication are February, April, June, August, October, and December. Business and Editorial Offices: 1600 John F. Kennedy Blvd., Suite 1800, Philadelphia, PA 19103-2899. Periodicals postage paid at New York, NY and additional mailing offices. Subscription prices are $370.00 per year for US individuals, $627.00 per year for US institutions, $180.00 per year for US students and residents, $455.00 per year for Canadian individuals, $793.00 per year for Canadian institutions, $510.00 for international individuals, $793.00 per year for international institutions and $250.00 per year for Canadian and foreign students/residents. To receive student/resident rate, orders must be accompanied by name of affiliated institution, date of term, and the *signature* of program/residency coordinator on institution letterhead. Orders will be billed at individual rate until proof of status is received. Foreign air speed delivery is included in all *Clinics* subscription prices. All prices are subject to change without notice. POSTMASTER: Send address changes to *Surgical Clinics*, Elsevier Health Sciences Division, Subscription Customer Service, 3251 Riverport Lane, Maryland Heights, MO 63043. **Customer Service (orders, claims, online, change of address): Telephone: 1-800-654-2452 (U.S. and Canada); 314-447-8871 (outside U.S. and Canada). Fax: 314-447-8029. E-mail: journalscustomerservice-usa@elsevier.com (for print support); journalsonline support-usa@elsevier.com (for online support).**

Reprints. For copies of 100 or more, of articles in this publication, please contact the Commercial Reprints Department, Elsevier Inc., 360 Park Avenue South, New York, New York 10010-1710. Tel. 212-633-3874, Fax: 212-633-3820, e-mail: reprints@elsevier.com.

The Surgical Clinics of North America is also published in Spanish by McGraw-Hill Interamericana Editores S.A., P.O. Box 5-237 06500 Mexico D.F. Mexico; and in Portuguese by Interlivros Edicoes Ltda., Rua Comandante Coelho 1085, CEP 21250, Rio de Janeiro, Brazil; and in Greek by Paschalidis Medical Publications, Athens Greece.

The Surgical Clinics of North America is covered in *MEDLINE/PubMed (Index Medicus)*, *EMBASE/Excerpta Medica*, *Current Contents/Clinical Medicine*, *Current Contents/Life Sciences*, *Science Citation Index*, and *ISI/BIOMED*.

Printed and bound by CPI Group (UK) Ltd, Croydon, CR0 4YY

Transferred to digital print 2013

Contributors

CONSULTING EDITOR

RONALD F. MARTIN, MD, FACS
Staff Surgeon, Department of Surgery, Marshfield Clinic, Marshfield; Clinical Associate Professor, University of Wisconsin School of Medicine and Public Health, Madison, Wisconsin; Colonel, Medical Corps, United States Army Reserve

EDITOR

GEORGE C. VELMAHOS, MD, PhD, MSEd
John F. Burke Professor of Surgery, Harvard Medical School; Chief of Trauma, Emergency Medicine, and Surgical Critical Care, Massachusetts General Hospital, Boston, Massachusetts

AUTHORS

HASAN B. ALAM, MD
Norman Thompson Professor of Surgery, Chief of General Surgery, Department of Surgery, University of Michigan Health System, Ann Arbor, Michigan

MITCHELL JAY COHEN, MD, FACS
Associate Professor of Surgery in Residence, Department of Surgery, Associate Trauma Medical Director, Director of Trauma Research, San Francisco General Hospital, University of California San Francisco, San Francisco, California

STEVEN R. DEMEESTER, MD
Professor, Department of Surgery, Keck School of Medicine, University of Southern California, Los Angeles, California

DEMETRIOS DEMETRIADES, MD, PhD
Professor of Surgery, Director, Division of Acute Care Surgery, University of Southern California, Los Angeles, California

MARC A. DE MOYA, MD
Assistant Professor of Surgery, Division of Trauma, Emergency Surgery, and Surgical Critical Care, Department of Surgery, Massachusetts General Hospital, Boston, Massachusetts

PETER J. FAGENHOLZ, MD
Division of Trauma, Emergency Surgery, and Surgical Critical Care, Department of Surgery, Massachusetts General Hospital, Boston; Instructor in Surgery, Harvard Medical School, Boston, Massachusetts

MARCIE FEINMAN, MD
Assistant in Surgery, Division of Acute Care Surgery, Department of Surgery, Anesthesiology/Critical Care Medicine (ACCM), Emergency Medicine, The Johns Hopkins University School of Medicine, Baltimore, Maryland

ELLIOTT R. HAUT, MD, FACS
Associate Professor of Surgery, Division of Acute Care Surgery, Department of Surgery, Anesthesiology/Critical Care Medicine (ACCM), Emergency Medicine, The Johns Hopkins University School of Medicine, Baltimore, Maryland

HAYTHAM M.A. KAAFARANI, MD, MPH
Division of Trauma, Emergency Surgery and Surgical Critical Care, Massachusetts General Hospital, Harvard Medical School, Boston, Massachusetts

GEORGE KASOTAKIS, MD, MPH
Assistant Professor of Surgery, Section of Trauma & Acute Care Surgery, Boston Medical Center, Boston University School of Medicine, Boston, Massachusetts

DAVID R. KING, MD
Division of Trauma, Emergency Surgery and Surgical Critical Care, Massachusetts General Hospital, Harvard Medical School, Boston, Massachusetts

RAMINDER NIRULA, MD, MPH
Associate Professor, Department of Surgery, University of Utah, Salt Lake City, Utah

ALI SALIM, MD, FACS
Chief, Division of Trauma, Burns, and Surgical Critical Care, Brigham and Women's Hospital; Lecturer in Surgery, Harvard Medical School, Boston, Massachusetts

MICHAEL J. SISE, MD, FACS
Clinical Professor, Department of Surgery, University of California San Diego School of Medicine; Medical Director, Division of Trauma, Scripps Mercy Hospital, San Diego, California

JASON SPERRY, MD, MPH, FACS
Associate Professor of Surgery and Critical Care, Associate Director of Acute Care Surgery Fellowship, University of Pittsburgh Medical Center, Pittsburgh, Pennsylvania

STEPHANIE G. WORRELL, MD
General Surgery Resident, Department of Surgery, Keck School of Medicine, University of Southern California, Los Angeles, California

D. DANTE YEH, MD
Clinical Instructor, Department of Surgery, Massachusetts General Hospital, Harvard Medical School, Boston, Massachusetts

Contents

> Infectious and inflammatory diseases comprise some of the most common gastrointestinal disorders resulting in hospitalization in the United States. Accordingly, they occupy a significant proportion of the workload of the acute care surgeon. This article discusses the diagnosis, management, and treatment of appendicitis, acute cholecystitis/cholangitis, acute pancreatitis, diverticulitis, and *Clostridium difficile* colitis.

> The cause and management of gastroduodenal perforation have changed as a result of increasing use of nonsteroidal antiinflammatories and improved pharmacologic treatment of acid hypersecretion as well as the recognition and treatment of *Helicobacter pylori*. As a result of the reduction in ulcer recurrence with medical therapy, the surgical approach to patients with gastroduodenal perforation has also changed over the last 3 decades, with ulcer-reducing surgery being performed infrequently.

> Esophageal perforation is uncommon but carries a high morbidity and mortality, particularly if the injury is not detected early before the onset of systemic signs of sepsis. The fact that it is an uncommon problem and it produces symptoms that can mimic other serious thoracic conditions, such as myocardial infarction, contributes to the delay in diagnosis. Patients at risk for iatrogenic perforations (esophageal malignancy) frequently have comorbidities that increase their perioperative morbidity and mortality. The optimal treatment of esophageal perforation varies with respect to the time of presentation, the extent of the perforation, and the underlying esophageal pathologic conditions.

> Upper gastrointestinal (GI) bleeding remains a commonly encountered diagnosis for acute care surgeons. Initial stabilization and resuscitation of patients is imperative. Stable patients can have initiation of medical therapy and localization of the bleeding, whereas persistently unstable

patients require emergent endoscopic or operative intervention. Minimally invasive techniques have surpassed surgery as the treatment of choice for most upper GI bleeding.

This article examines causes of occult, moderate and severe lower gastrointestinal (GI) bleeding. The difference in the workup of stable vs unstable patients is stressed. Treatment options ranging from minimally invasive techniques to open surgery are explored.

Spontaneous hemoperitoneum is a rare, but life-threatening condition usually caused by nontraumatic rupture of the liver, spleen, or abdominal vasculature with underlying pathology. Management revolves around angioembolization or surgical intervention. This article provides a brief overview of the diagnosis and treatment of this disorder.

The retroperitoneum is rich in vascular structures and can harbor large hematomas, traumatic or spontaneous. The management of retroperitoneal hematomas depends on the mechanism of injury and whether they are pulsatile/expanding. Rectus sheath hematomas are uncommon abdominal wall hematomas secondary to trauma to the epigastric arteries of the rectus muscle. The common risk factors include anticoagulation, strenuous exercise, coughing, coagulation disorders, and invasive procedures on/ through the abdominal wall. The management is largely supportive, with the reversal of anticoagulation and transfusions; angioembolization may be necessary.

Acute obstruction of the gastrointestinal or biliary tract represents a common problem for acute care surgeons. It is with appropriate clinical evaluation, planning, and physical examination follow-up that acute care surgeons are able to appropriately diagnose, manage, and resolve this difficult group of surgical problems and minimize the morbidity associated with each.

Hernia emergencies are commonly encountered by the acute care surgeon. Although the location and contents may vary, the basic principles are constant: address the life-threatening problem first, then perform the safest and most durable hernia repair possible. Mesh reinforcement provides the most durable long-term results. Underlay positioning is associated with the best outcomes. Components separation is a useful technique to achieve tension-free primary fascial reapproximation. The choice of mesh is dictated by the degree of contamination. Internal herniation is rare, and preoperative diagnosis remains difficult. In all hernia emergencies, morbidity is high, and postoperative wound complications should be anticipated.

The open abdomen has become the standard of care in damage-control procedures, the management of intra-abdominal hypertension, and in severe intra-abdominal sepsis. This approach has saved many lives but has also created new problems, such as severe fluid and protein loss, nutritional problems, enteroatmospheric fistulas, fascial retraction with loss of abdominal domain, and development of massive incisional hernias. Early definitive closure is the basis of preventing or reducing the risk of these complications. The introduction of new techniques and materials for temporary and subsequent definitive abdominal closure has improved outcomes in this group of patients.

Necrotizing skin and soft tissue infections are severe bacterial infections resulting in rapid and life-threatening soft tissue destruction and necrosis along soft tissue planes.

Acute mesenteric ischemia is uncommon and always occurs in the setting of preexisting comorbidities. Mortality rates remain high. The 4 major types of acute mesenteric ischemia are acute superior mesenteric artery thromboembolic occlusion, mesenteric arterial thrombosis, mesenteric venous thrombosis, and nonocclusive mesenteric ischemia, including ischemic colitis. Delays in diagnosis are common and associated with high rates of morbidity and mortality. Prompt diagnosis requires attention to history and physical examination, a high index of suspicion, and early contract CT scanning. Selective use of nonoperative therapy has an important role in nonocclusive mesenteric ischemia of the small bowel and colon.

This article discusses thoracic emergencies, including the anatomy, pathophysiology, clinical presentation, examination, diagnosis, technique, management, and treatment of acute upper airway obstruction, massive hemoptysis, spontaneous pneumothorax, and pulmonary empyema.

SURGICAL CLINICS
OF NORTH AMERICA

FORTHCOMING ISSUES

April 2014
Biliary Tract Surgery
Jessica A. Wernberg, MD, *Editor*

June 2014
Endocrine Surgery
Peter J. Mazzaglia, MD, *Editor*

August 2014
Management of Burns
Robert Sheridan, MD, *Editor*

RECENT ISSUES

December 2013
Current Topics in Transplantation
A. Osama Gaber, MD, *Editor*

October 2013
Abdominal Wall Reconstruction
Michael J. Rosen, MD, *Editor*

August 2013
Vascular Surgery and Endovascular Therapy
Girma Tefera, MD, *Editor*

June 2013
Modern Concepts in Pancreatic Surgery
Stephen W. Behrman, MD, FACS, and
Ronald F. Martin, MD, FACS, *Editors*

ISSUE OF RELATED INTEREST

Emergency Medicine Clinics of North America February 2013 (Vol. 31, Issue 1)
Critical Skills and Procedures in Emergency Medicine
Jorge L. Falcon-Chevere, MD, and Jose G. Cabanas, MD, *Editors*

NOW AVAILABLE FOR YOUR iPhone and iPad

Foreword

Acute Care Surgery

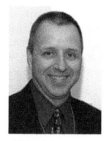

Ronald F. Martin, MD, FACS
Consulting Editor

For the readers of the *Surgical Clinics of North America* who have had the opportunity to glance at the forewords I have previously written, it should come as no surprise that I struggle with the concept of General Surgery. In large part that is why I agreed to be the Consulting Editor of this series: I thought it would help me answer the question of what a general surgeon was. Nearly a decade later, and with the help of some very thoughtful and intelligent people, I am not sure I am much closer to understanding.

In fact, the more things change and the more I study this, I think I get more confused.

This issue of the *Surgical Clinics of North America* is devoted to Acute Care Surgery. Even the term acute care surgery doesn't make sense to me. Mind you, I know how we use it—any surgical problem in a patient that requires our attention that is not accompanied by the patient making a scheduled appointment—but that is not super helpful to me. After all, who ever stated that "regular surgery" was the discipline of taking care of people with surgical problems who presented by way of an appointment? Is "acute care surgery" just a euphemism for problems that come to our notice at an inconvenient time?

I recently attended a panel session at the American College of Surgeons Clinical Congress in Washington, DC. As with all major panel sessions at the College (excepting any I might serve on) the panelists are famous leaders in the field. I won't mention the names of the panelists but what struck me about the group was the vintage. A little biographical investigation later I determined that each participant was in his (and they were all males) 60s and the majority closer to 70 than 60. These guys are absolutely the big dogs of the game and it was fun to watch them spar with one another in front of the crowd. Yet, I couldn't get over the fact that they all missed the most fundamental point there is—we don't and won't make new surgeons like them anymore. Period. Not going to happen, moving on now.

All of these surgeons trained before computed tomography, magnetic resonance, even ultrasonography. Some of them predate out-of-operating room mechanical ventilation. All of them predate work hours restrictions and probably all trained in the era of

http://dx.doi.org/10.1016/j.suc.2013.10.015
0039-6109/14/$ – see front matter © 2014 Elsevier Inc. All rights reserved.
surgical.theclinics.com

pyramidal residency programs. As a program director in surgery, I could not try to replicate their training environment without losing my residency program, possibly my institutional accreditation, and definitely my job. Even some of the cases that were presented were old chestnuts long since kept on the shelf for just such an occasion as this panel. When one of the panelists asked why the presenter did not order a CT scan for a particular patient, the presenter finally confessed it was because the case under discussion occurred before the advent of CT scanning. In short, all of these panelists trained when we knew what general surgery was because there was almost nothing else to confuse it with. Everybody did most everything and everybody was always around to see how things went, poorly or well. These panelists have worked in that model their entire professional lives.

Over the years since their training, trauma and critical care have coalesced and separated themselves away from general surgery in most environments. Also, over the years, trauma, in particular blunt trauma, has bordered on a nonoperative discipline. This trend has been pretty steady for the past 25 to 30 years. It may be possible as well, though I cannot remotely prove this, that some people have sought further training, or have been counseled to do so, in trauma and critical care specifically because of the tilt toward a more nonoperative specialty. In recent years, the diminished level of operative activity of many "trauma surgeons" became a major concern of trauma center verifiers and led many trauma programs to find ways to increase their surgeon operative exposure. This need, coupled with a markedly diminished appetite of other surgeons to come to work in the middle of the night, made the "acute care surgery" service and the "trauma" service a natural schedule fit—after all, neither patient thinks to make an appointment.

In the meantime, though, specialization of almost everything that was general surgery had already happened. Breast, foregut, hindgut, thoracic, vascular, endocrine, oncology, and more had all become islands of their own to some degree. Each of these specialties had also raised the bar of performance.

So now we have a group of patients being cared for by surgeons who are most available rather than necessarily the most capable surgeons, and maybe that's okay. It is better to have a possibly somewhat less trained person to help when you need it in a hurry than to have an expert who can see you when your situation is irretrievable. Still, I struggle with idea that one develops nocturnal excellence or weekend excellence across the entire spectrum of general surgery.

No matter how we got here or how we feel about where we are: here we are and we are not going back. So the question becomes: will the acute care surgery model be the rebirth of general surgery as we knew it or will it be the final dissolution of the general surgeon into a series of subunits?

Personally, I bet on neither.

There are some factors we can probably rely on as we move forward. Society wants and will demand that we will do more for less and with less. Also, they will demand that we do that better than we have historically. If I am remotely correct on this, then the separation of acute care surgery from subspecialty surgery will be a nonstarter. We will have to work in teams; we will have to share responsibility and collaborate. If we don't, we will likely use resources less wisely and unnecessarily damage the innocents. The costs for suboptimal management and care will come out of our hides by way of reputation and financially. Devising systems in which we balance who takes point and who is ready to join in on short notice for exceptional challenges will likely be more efficient and more effective. Finding ways to balance continuity needs and 24/7 availability of surgeons who are not falling asleep will be required. The main barriers are financial and, for lack of a better term, surgeon-ego. Altered compensation schemes are easy enough to devise as are working solutions to the physician-centric complaints, though they are monumentally hard to get people to buy into them. Maintaining a patient-centric or even a patient-community-centric model will be required and is achievable.

Regardless of whether one thinks that the development of acute care is a great advancement and restoration of general surgery or represents the final nail in the coffin of general surgery—it probably lies in between those extremes—one should not argue with the notion that the more one knows about the kinds of problems and solutions required for patients who show up unexpectedly ill, the better off everybody will be. Dr Velmahos and his colleagues have done a wonderful job of collecting wisdom that will serve us all. I encourage all to consider their writings well.

Ronald F. Martin, MD, FACS
Department of Surgery
Marshfield Clinic
1000 North Oak Avenue
Marshfield, WI 54449, USA

E-mail address:
martin.ronald@marshfieldclinic.org

Preface

Acute Care Surgery: From De Novo to De Facto

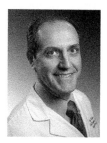

George C. Velmahos, MD, PhD, MSEd
Editor

There is little debate anymore about the need for Acute Care Surgery (ACS). It seems like yesterday—and it is indeed less than 10 years ago—that general surgeons, trauma surgeons, neurosurgeons, orthopedic surgeons, and administrators alike were entangled in confusing and often contradicting arguments about ACS. Like every change, this particular one was not to be accepted without resistance and disbelief. Eventually, it was put to the unmistaken test of public use. It was tried in various hospitals and left to succeed or fail according to its ability to improve the process and outcomes of care. Now, in 2014, as most hospitals around the country have developed or are in the process of developing ACS programs, we can confirm that the model was a success.

The need for ACS was born out of the discrepancy between the care delivered to trauma and nontrauma emergency patients. Over nearly five decades, our country developed an enviable system for the care of the injured. Trauma teams, trauma centers, and trauma protocols were created to ensure that trauma patients are managed in an organized and comprehensive manner. Regionalization of trauma care allowed interconnectivity between centers, delivery of patients to the right place according to resources and commitment, and transfer of care from lower to higher levels of trauma centers, when the need arises. The American College of Surgeons directed and supported this effort in numerous ways through its Committee on Trauma. None of these existed for nontraumatic surgical emergencies. Unlike trauma, the care provided to patients with a surgical disease of nontraumatic cause was often fragmented and possibly inadequate. There were no dedicated teams and no well-planned systems for these patients who arrived in the middle of the night with a perforated diverticulum, a bleeding ulcer, or an obstructed bowel.

To complicate things further, the increasing trend of subspecialization among US surgical residency graduates was leaving a huge void in call coverage. Particularly in tertiary centers, surgeons had become masters of one specific body region or even one specific organ. Often by mandate from the institution, they were focused on the

Surg Clin N Am 94 (2014) xiii–xv
http://dx.doi.org/10.1016/j.suc.2013.10.014
0039-6109/14/$ – see front matter © 2014 Elsevier Inc. All rights reserved.
surgical.theclinics.com

practice of breast, endocrine, colorectal, foregut, or pancreatobiliary surgery. When night came, they were asked to revert to broad-based general surgery and, as a matter of fact, under the most adverse conditions on the most unstable patients. It was not always easy, particularly when a full elective operative schedule or clinic was waiting the next morning. Nontraumatic emergency surgical disease was not always managed in the best possible way or by the most qualified person. As a young trauma surgeon, I can vividly remember the trauma bay bustling with the activities of our robust trauma team, spread around the bed of a patient with critical injuries. Too many people in the room was the typical problem. In the next bay, a patient with peritonitis and sepsis received only a fraction of this activity and often in the absence of a surgical team. The room was often quite empty.

Following deliberations with multiple interested stakeholders, the American Association for the Surgery of Trauma established in 2003 the ad-hoc Committee to Develop the Re-organized Specialty of Trauma, Surgical Critical Care, and Emergency Surgery.[1] Eventually, this became the standing Acute Care Surgery Committee and led the effort of developing a curriculum for ACS fellowship and defining the scope of practice of ACS.[2] With the understanding that one size does not fit all, the leaders of this effort balanced the need for standardization with the flexibility to conform to local standards. Initially, a few academic institutions explored the benefits of an ACS team. Based on early positive feedback, more institutions followed and quite rapidly the concept spread in academia and community practice alike. I can remember only a few examples of explosive expansion of a new concept in my career and ACS is one of them. From a debated and mistrusted novelty it became a fact of surgical practice within only a few years.

No doubt exists that there is a lot of work to be done. The initial intent of including orthopedic and neurosurgical procedures in the ACS surgeon's gamut was met with resistance by the relevant subspecialty societies, and to a great extent, abandoned.[3,4] The overlap with the general surgeon's practice is still significant. The boundaries of ACS need to be refined according to the basic rule of delivering care to the right person at the right place at the right time (by the right surgeons, I might add). Different institutions have different needs. We should allow the flexibility to apply slightly different ACS models in academic versus community hospitals and in large versus small centers. Training goals and methods must be better defined.

We have come a long distance. ACS now encompasses trauma, surgical critical care, and emergency nontraumatic surgery.[5] The scope of practice in emergency surgery is increasingly understood. For me it is defined by four simple words: bleeding, obstruction, perforation, and inflammation (acute). The American Association for the Surgery of Trauma has described it in greater detail by a list of relevant ICD-9 codes.[6] There are 16 ACS fellowship programs that produce trained and committed ACS surgeons every year. Many more are prepared to follow. The training in general surgery has been enhanced after the creation of ACS teams.[7] Academic scholarship on ACS is ramping up and the trauma community, which has traditionally excelled in the research of injury and resuscitation, is applying its research infrastructure in emergency surgical diseases.[8] Finances improve, and departments with ACS teams have realized increased revenues at the ACS division without compromising the profit of general surgeons.[9] Quality control and productivity initiatives from the well-oiled trauma QA machine have fertilized the emergency nontraumatic surgery world.[10,11] Finally, not to be minimized, the perceptions of young trainees, who were recently ranking trauma surgery low in their preferences, have now changed and ACS is considered a desirable career goal.[12]

With all this in mind, the current issue of the *Surgical Clinics of North America* presents a compilation of nontraumatic emergency surgery diseases that are frequently managed by ACS teams. Most of them are confined to the abdomen. Some are extra-abdominal and universally within the purview of the ACS surgeon (eg, necrotizing fasciitis). Others depend on local standards, expertise, and culture (eg, thoracic or vascular emergencies). The collaboration with subspecialists should only be viewed in a positive light as a way to enhance patient care, never as a turf war. The ACS model should be based on inclusion not exclusion. The experts who authored the articles are nationally recognized authorities, who have devoted their professional lives to the care of the patient in need. They write from experience, knowledge, and the heart.

George C. Velmahos, MD, PhD, MSEd
Massachusetts General Hospital
Harvard Medical School
165 Cambridge Street, Suite 810
Boston, MA 02114, USA

E-mail address:
gvelmahos@partners.org

REFERENCES

1. Committee to Develop the Reorganized Specialty of Trauma Surgical Critical Care and Emergency Surgery. Acute care surgery: trauma, critical care, and emergency surgery. J Trauma 2005;58:614–6.
2. The Acute Care Surgery Committee of the American Association for the Surgery of Trauma. The Acute Care Surgery curriculum. J Trauma 2007;62:553–6.
3. Vrahas MS. Acute care surgery from the orthopedic surgeon's perspective: a lost opportunity. Surgery 2007;141:317–20.
4. Byrne RW, Bagan BT, Bingaman W, et al. Emergency neurosurgical care solutions: Acute Care Surgery, regionalization, and the neurosurgeon: results of the 2008 CNS consensus sessions. Neurosurgery 2011;68:1063–7.
5. Velmahos GC, Jurkovich JG. The concept of Acute Care Surgery: a vision for the not-so-distant future. Surgery 2007;141:288–9.
6. Shafi S, Aboutanos M, Agarwal S Jr, et al. Emergency general surgery: definition and estimated burden of disease. J Trauma Acute Care Surg 2013;74:1092–7.
7. Stanley MD, Davenport DL, Procter LD, et al. An Acute Care Surgery rotation contributes significant general surgical operative volume to residency training compared to other rotations. J Trauma 2011;70:590–4.
8. Early BJ, Huang DT, Callaway CW, et al. Multidisciplinary acute care research organization (MACRO): if you build it, they will come. J Trauma Acute Care Surg 2013;75:106–9.
9. Miller PR, Wildman EA, Chang MC, et al. Acute care surgery: impact on practice and economics of elective surgeons. J Am Coll Surg 2012;214:531–5.
10. Barnes SL, Cooper CJ, Coughenour JP, et al. Impact of acute care surgery to departmental productivity. J Trauma 2011;71:1027–32.
11. Ingraham AM, Haas B, Cohen ME, et al. Comparison of hospital performance in trauma vs. emergency and elective general surgery. Arch Surg 2012;147:591–8.
12. Moore HB, Moore PK, Grant AR, et al. Future of acute care surgery: a perspective from the next generation. J Trauma 2012;72:94–9.

Acute Inflammatory Surgical Disease

Peter J. Fagenholz, MD*, Marc A. de Moya, MD

KEYWORDS

- Appendicitis • Cholecystitis • Cholangitis • Pancreatitis • Diverticulitis
- Clostridium difficile • Colitis

KEY POINTS

- Computed tomography is the most accurate way to diagnose appendicitis and its complications. Abscesses should be percutaneously drained, phlegmon treated with antibiotics, and appendectomy performed in most other cases.
- Immediate laparoscopic cholecystectomy is standard treatment for acute cholecystitis, though percutaneous cholecystostomy is effective in high risk patients. Cholangitis should be treated with endoscopic retrograde cholangiography and sphincterotomy.
- Infected pancreatic necrosis is the primary indication for intervention in pancreatitis. A "step-up" approach beginning with percutaneous or endoscopic drainage and proceeding to surgical debridement when necessary should be used.
- Diverticulitis without abscess or with small abscess should be treated with antibiotics alone. Large diverticular abscesses should be percutaneously drained. In cases of free perforation with peritonitis mandating surgery, primary anastomosis with or without proximal diversion should be considered.
- Subtotal colectomy with end ileostomy is standard surgical therapy for medically refractory Clostridium difficile colitis. There may be a role for ileostomy with antegrade colonic lavage.

Infectious and inflammatory diseases comprise some of the most common gastrointestinal disorders resulting in hospitalization in the United States. Accordingly, they occupy a significant proportion of the workload of the acute care surgeon.

Disclosures: Neither of the authors have any relevant conflicts of interest to disclose.
Division of Trauma, Emergency Surgery, and Surgical Critical Care, Department of Surgery, Massachusetts General Hospital, 165 Cambridge Street, CPZ 810, Boston, MA 02114, USA
* Corresponding author.
E-mail address: pfagenholz@partners.org

http://dx.doi.org/10.1016/j.suc.2013.10.008
0039-6109/14/$ – see front matter © 2014 Elsevier Inc. All rights reserved.
surgical.theclinics.com

APPENDICITIS

> **Key points**
> - Young men with a typical clinical presentation do not require imaging.
> - Computed tomography with intravenous contrast is the imaging modality of choice when required.
> - Perforated appendicitis with abscess should be treated with percutaneous drainage.
> - Perforated appendicitis with phlegmon should be treated with antibiotics alone.
> - Laparoscopic appendectomy results in fewer surgical infections than open appendectomy.

In 1886, Reginald Fitz of Boston, in his monograph "Diseases of the Vermiform Appendix," correctly identified the appendix as the primary cause of right lower quadrant inflammation and coined the term appendicitis. Appendicitis is the most common problem of the colon, affecting approximately 300,000 patients a year and some estimate 8% of the Western country population will face appendicitis some time in their lives.[1] In the past, reliance on physical examination and laboratory findings have been the mainstay of diagnosis but in the era of computed tomography and ultrasound imaging, studies are increasingly accepted to assess for appendicitis. The standard treatment has traditionally been open appendectomy, but the number of laparoscopic appendectomies has now surpassed the number of open appendectomies in the United States. Even more recently, there has been a growing debate regarding the nonoperative approach to appendicitis, namely treatment with antibiotics. We review the basic diagnostic options and describe treatment options for acute appendicitis, including the treatment of the perforated appendicitis or delayed presentations.

Clinical History and Physical Examination

Appendicitis typically occurs as a result of the obstruction of the appendiceal lumen that subsequently results in ischemia and inflammation. This ischemia and inflammation evolves over several hours and is the cause of early visceral pain that then localizes to the right lower quadrant. The obstruction is typically the result of a fecolith or adenitis.[2] These processes lead to necrosis and perforation of the appendix, which occur usually after at least 48 hours of symptoms. The bacteriology of appendicitis is a mixed enteral flora, including *Escherichia coli*, *Streptococcus viridans*, and *Bacteroides* species.

The clinical history of appendicitis typically includes a 24-hour to 48-hour progression of vague periumbilical pain that migrates and becomes more localized to the right lower quadrant. The tenderness is usually a localized peritonitis with additional manifestations of pain on coughing (Dunphy sign), pain with flexion and internal rotation of the right hip (obturator sign), pain with passive extension of the right hip (psoas sign), or pain in the right lower quadrant during palpation of the left lower quadrant (Rovsing sign). In addition, patients may have tenderness with rectal examination.

The typical laboratory findings include a mild to moderate leukocytosis with a left shift, a urinalysis showing a few white blood cells, and other laboratory findings of inflammation, such as elevated C-reactive protein. The differential diagnosis of right lower quadrant tenderness includes sigmoid diverticulitis (secondary to a redundant sigmoid that reaches across the midline), cecal diverticulitis, retroperitoneal or rectus sheath hematoma, viral enteritis, Crohn disease, perforating colonic carcinoma, and, in women, a number of gynecologic pathologies. A meta-analysis done by Andersen[3] found that the history of migration of pain, peritoneal irritation, and elevated laboratory findings suggestive of an inflammatory process were the great predictors of appendicitis. Despite the history, physical findings, and laboratory findings, it is clear that there is no single confirmatory test. The use of physical examination, history, and laboratory values has in the past resulted in negative appendectomy rates of about 15%. One study also attributed $740 million in hospital charges in the 1990s to negative appendectomies.[4] As a result, a number of scoring systems have been developed to improve the positive predictive value of a combination of factors.

The most commonly used and referenced is the Alvarado or MANTRELS scoring system (**Table 1**).[5] Although the ability of the score, which is a compilation of multiple signs, symptoms, and laboratory values, is better than any individual piece of data, it does not have the power to reliably rule in or rule out appendicitis by itself. A score of 7 to 10 warrants appendectomy and those less than 7 are observed. Using this scoring system, there remains an 11% negative appendectomy rate, albeit improved from the 15% rate that is typical without using the score.

Radiographic Imaging

The continued evolution of ultrasound and computed tomography (CT) technology has significantly improved the sensitivity and specificity. Ultrasonography in adults has a sensitivity of approximately 83% with a specificity of approximately 93%. CT scan has a sensitivity of approximately 94% with a 94% specificity.[6] Therefore, whether to use either ultrasonography or CT to rule in or rule out the diagnosis is now an important consideration. The downside to CT is the ionizing energy and cost. The current recommendations of the Surgical Infection Society and Infectious Disease Society of America guidelines is to obtain helical CT with intravenous (IV) contrast as the test of choice when imaging is necessary.[7] Oral and rectal contrast are not necessary components of the imaging. The use of CT scanning has reduced negative appendectomy rates further to approximately 2.6%.[8] A proposed diagnostic algorithm is depicted in **Fig. 1**.

Treatment

Once the diagnosis of appendicitis is made, there are a few options for treatment: (1) appendectomy (open vs laparoscopic), (2) antibiotics, and (3) percutaneous drainage and antibiotics. The open appendectomy, first described by McBurney in 1889,[9] is a classic approach to appendicitis but has for the most part been replaced in the United

Table 1 Alvarado score		
	Variable	**Value**
Symptoms	Migration	1
	Anorexia	1
	Nausea-vomiting	1
Signs	Tenderness in right left quadrant	2
	Rebound tenderness	1
	Fever	1
Laboratory Values	White blood cells >10,000/µL	2
	Shift to the left (>75% neutrophils)	1
Total Score		10

Adapted from Alvarado A. A practical score for the early diagnosis of acute appendicitis. Ann Emerg Med 1986;15:557–64.

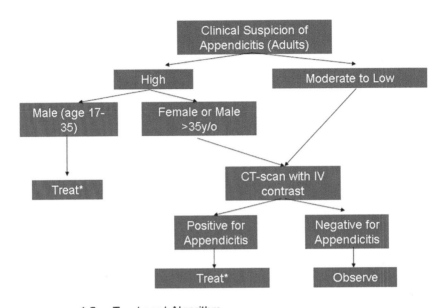

* See Treatment Algorithm

Fig. 1. Algorithm for diagnosis of acute appendicitis. y/o, years old.

States by laparoscopic appendectomy, first described by Semm in 1983.[10] In 2010, Ingraham and others[11] conducted a study using the American College of Surgeons National Surgical Quality Improvement Program across 222 hospitals. This study found that 76.4% of appendectomies were performed laparoscopically. Overall morbidity and surgical site infections were significantly lower in those who underwent laparoscopic surgery. Although this study supported the use of laparoscopic surgery, there were differences among the groups and they were not randomized. There are a number of randomized trials and in 2010 an update of a Cochrane meta-analysis found that the methodology in the randomized trials was moderate to poor but that there was an increased intra-abdominal infection with laparoscopic appendectomy, whereas open appendectomy had an increased risk of incisional infections. Overall, there is a decreased incidence of surgical infections using the laparoscopic approach; however, given the lack of definitive data, the open technique is still a viable option.

Although the surgical dictum since 1889 has been to remove the inflamed appendix, other inflammatory intra-abdominal processes, such as diverticulitis, have been increasingly treated with antibiotics rather than surgery. There is no question that there are complications associated with surgery for appendicitis and that resolution without surgery has been described. This has led some to consider more routine treatment of appendicitis with antibiotics. In 2006, Styrud and colleagues[12] undertook a randomized controlled trial to evaluate antibiotic treatment versus appendectomy. In 6 hospitals in Sweden they randomized 252 male patients to either antibiotic treatment (2 g IV cefotaxime twice a day for 2 days and 0.8 g tinidazole once daily followed by 10 days of oral ofloxacin) versus appendectomy (open or laparoscopic). Of the 128 randomized to antibiotics, 85% were successfully treated without surgery; 18 of the 128 were operated on within 24 hours and all but one had an acute appendicitis. There were no differences in the number of perforated appendicitis between the 2 groups. The rate of recurrence of symptoms was 14% during the 1-year follow-up. Since then, a follow-up study in Sweden randomized 369 male and female unselected patients to antibiotics versus surgery, which also demonstrated a 14% recurrence rate at 1 year.[13] Efficacy of antibiotic treatment was 90%.

In those patients who present with an appendiceal abscess, the diagnosis is confirmed with CT scan and treatment is typically with a percutaneously placed drain and antibiotics. A number of studies comparing early appendectomy to percutaneous drainage and antibiotic treatment in the setting of appendiceal abscess have favored percutaneous drainage and antibiotics. A treatment algorithm is proposed in **Fig. 2**.

ACUTE CHOLECYSTITIS/CHOLANGITIS

Key points

- Immediate cholecystectomy is the treatment of choice for acute cholecystitis.
- Cholecystostomy tube is a very effective option for poor-risk patients.
- Immediate endoscopic retrograde cholangiopancreatography (ERCP) is the preferred treatment for cholangitis.

Acute cholecystitis is the most common inflammatory process of the biliary tree, occurring in 20% to 30% of patients with symptomatic biliary colic. The inflammatory process may be calculous or acalculous in origin, most commonly calculous. It is estimated that 20 million people are diagnosed with gallstones, with more than a million hospitalizations and 700,000 operative procedures per year.[14] By the age of 70, 15% of men and 24% of women have gallstones, and this number increases to 24% and 35%, respectively, by the age of 90.[15,16] However, two-thirds of those with gallstones are asymptomatic.[17] The risk of becoming symptomatic is approximately 1% to 4% per year.[18] Calculous cholecystitis is caused by the acute obstruction of the cystic duct by a gallstone. Acalculous cholecystitis is an inflammatory process that is related to stasis and dysfunction of the gallbladder and is most commonly associated with a systemic critical illness.

Calculous Acute Cholecystitis

Once the cystic duct is obstructed, patients present with increasing right upper quadrant pain that often migrates from the epigastrium. This pain may be associated with

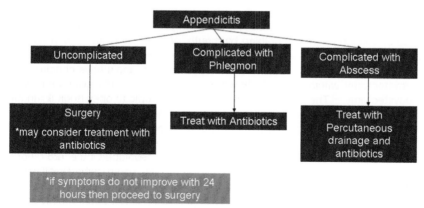

Fig. 2. Algorithm for treatment of acute appendicitis.

nausea and vomiting, fever, and malaise. On physical examination the patient will demonstrate right upper quadrant tenderness, which may include a Murphy sign. The Murphy sign is tenderness on inspiration with palpation overlying the gallbladder that causes the patient to arrest their attempt at a full inspiration. It is uncommon for patients to become jaundiced, but they may present with mild jaundice. Often this mild obstructive pattern is the result of a partial obstruction of the right hepatic duct or common bile duct by the inflamed gallbladder (Mirizzi syndrome).[19] Typical laboratory values include a moderately elevated white blood cell count in the range of 10 to 17 cells/mm^3, mild elevation of total bilirubin, alkaline phosphatase, transaminases, or amylase.[6]

The diagnosis is usually made by the combination of history, physical examination, and laboratory findings; however, imaging provides important additional information. The most helpful initial imaging study is the ultrasound of the right upper quadrant. This study provides the surgeon with evidence of cholelithiasis with a sensitivity and specificity greater than 95%.[5,20] It can also demonstrate ultrasonographic signs of acute cholecystitis, including a thickened gallbladder wall (>4 mm), pericholecystic fluid, and a sonographic Murphy sign (more sensitive than the traditional Murphy sign because the probe can be accurately applied directly to the gallbladder). A positive ultrasonic Murphy sign has a sensitivity and specificity of approximately 85% to 95% for acute cholecystitis. This study also provides information regarding the size of the common bile duct (normal <8 mm), although the sensitivity for gall-stones in the common bile duct is low due to overlying duodenal air. A hepatobiliary iminodiacetic acid scan is the use of radiotracer that is excreted in the bile. This study is a functional one and will demonstrate a lack of bile flow into the gallbladder, which is suggestive of an obstructed cystic duct; however, this test is not the first-line test for acute cholecystitis due to lack of wide rapid availability and cost.[21] The role of CT scan is limited but may be used in cases in which the ultrasound, serum tests, history, and physical are equivocal and to assess for other potential causes of abdominal pain when the diagnosis is unclear.

The duration of the obstruction and inflammation is related to the severity of gall-bladder wall ischemia. The ischemia leads to the spectrum of disease ranging from inflammation, purulent cholecystitis gallbladder, emphysematous gallbladder, to frank necrosis (**Fig. 3**) and perforation. The gallbladder may become secondarily infected as a result of the stasis of bile with *E coli* and *Klebsiella* being the most common organisms.

Treatment

Treatment of acute calculus cholecystitis is supportive with a nasogastric tube if nausea or vomiting persists, nothing by mouth, IV fluids, antibiotics, and cholecys-tectomy (laparoscopic or open). The timing of the cholecystectomy has drawn some debate over the years, but a few randomized controlled trials have concluded that cholecystectomy within 24 to 72 hours is advantageous compared with delayed cholecystectomy.[22] The conversion rate from laparoscopic to open is similar in these patients and the complication rate is lower in the immediate cholecystectomy groups. Therefore, it is generally recommended to perform a cholecystectomy within 24 hours of the patient's admission. During this time period, the laparoscopic cho-lecystectomy is occasionally made easier by planes developed by edema. For pa-tients presenting with 5 or more days of symptoms, some debate still remains whether immediate cholecystectomy is appropriate or is associated with high rates of open conversion and complications. This question has not been directly studied. If the patient is deemed not a surgical candidate, then the gallbladder may be

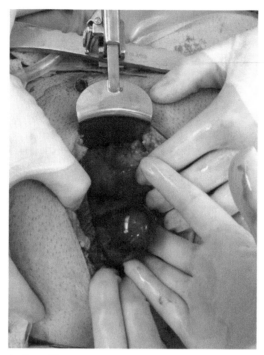

Fig. 3. Necrotizing cholecystitis.

percutaneously drained. Percutaneous drainage is more than 90% effective and patients usually improve within 24 hours after drainage. If improvement has not occurred by 24 hours, then one may consider the possibility of medical failure and may have to revert to cholecystectomy. The role and timing of percutaneous cholecystostomy has not been clearly defined according to a recent meta-analysis.[23] However, it is clear that particularly in the high-risk elderly that it is an effective and at times definitive treatment.[24] The timing of, need for, and optimal technique for interval cholecystectomy after percutaneous cholecystostomy tube placement has not been definitively studied. We typically perform cholecystostomy tube injection 4 to 6 weeks after drainage. If tube injection shows a persistently occluded cystic duct, we recommend cholecystectomy in all but the most medically infirm patients. If the cystic duct is patent, the risks and benefits of cholecystectomy can be determined on a case-by-case basis. A complete algorithm for management of acute cholecystitis is provided in **Fig. 4**.

Acalculous Cholecystitis

Only 5% to 10% of all cases of cholecystitis are acalculous. The symptoms are similar to calculous cholecystitis but usually occur in the face of concomitant critical illness. The illness may be medical or traumatic. An underlying sepsis or state of shock is often associated with acalculous cholecystitis and, therefore, early treatment with antibiotics and an intervention are warranted. Most cases are treated with percutaneous cholecystostomy but cholecystectomy is an option. The mortality rate for this condition may be up to 40% because of the associated comorbid conditions.

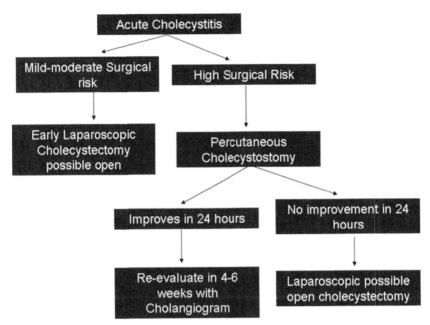

Fig. 4. Algorithm for treatment of acute cholecystitis.

Acute Cholangitis

Acute cholangitis is the result of 2 forces: obstruction and bacterbilia. The bacterbilia is thought be a result of biliary stasis and obstruction. The obstruction causes acute elevations in the biliary pressures leading to rapid bacteremia and sepsis. The 3 typical features of cholangitis (fever, jaundice, and right upper quadrant pain) were described in 1877 by Charcot. The most common cause of obstruction is gallstones; however, benign and malignant strictures, instrumentation, or periampullary cancer have also caused cholangitis.[6]

Patients will present with Charcot triad (described previously); however, severe disease is often accompanied by hypotension and change in mental status with these 5 signs termed Reynold pentad. Fever, often with rigors, is the commonest sign. The laboratory findings are what one might find with a septic patient with an elevated white blood cell count and a left shift. In addition, given the biliary obstruction responsible for the disease, the total bilirubin levels will be elevated with most being direct bilirubinemia along with associated elevations in alkaline phosphatases and transaminases.

Once the diagnosis is made, treatment is initiated immediately with antibiotic administration and fluid resuscitation. An ERCP is performed with stone extraction and sphincterotomy. If the patient presents with severe symptoms, an emergent ERCP is indicated.[25] If the ampulla cannot be cannulated, then a percutaneous transhepatic cholangiocatheter (PTC) may be performed[26] or surgical decompression. ERCP and PTC are less invasive and therefore are the preferred approach in these often unstable patients.[27] Those patients who recover uneventfully should undergo a cholecystectomy if they are not prohibitive surgical candidates. With sphincterotomy, the recurrence rate of biliary complications is decreased from 25% to 5% and therefore may be considered all that is required in patients with multiple other comorbidities.[28,29]

ACUTE PANCREATITIS

Key points

- Imaging is rarely needed to diagnose acute pancreatitis and should not generally be performed at presentation.

- CT scanning with intravenous contrast should be performed to assess for local complications in patients failing to improve.

- Infected necrosis is the most common indication for surgery in acute pancreatitis, but intervention should be delayed for 4 weeks whenever possible.

- Minimally invasive percutaneous or endoscopic drainage should be the first intervention in infected necrotizing pancreatitis.

- If minimally invasive drainage does not resolve the infected necrosis, surgical debridement is needed.

Acute pancreatitis encompasses a wide range of severity, from mild and self-limited to lethal. In its severe forms, the disease tests the judgment, patience, and tenacity of even the most experienced surgeons. This section answers the most common clinical questions related to care of acute pancreatitis, such as which patients should receive antibiotics, what is the best method of nutrition, which patients require surgery, what is the optimal surgical approach, and others.

Epidemiology and Etiology

Acute pancreatitis is the most common gastrointestinal disorder requiring hospitalization in the United States, with an estimated 274,000 hospitalizations in 2009 and its incidence appears to be increasing.[30,31] In the United States, cases are evenly distributed between men and women, although alcohol is more commonly the cause in men and gallstones are more commonly the cause in women. The incidence increases with increasing age, although the greatest number of cases occur in patients in the fifth or sixth decade of life.[30] The most common causes of acute pancreatitis are ethanol ingestion and gallstones. Less frequent causes include instrumentation of the bile or pancreatic ducts (ERCP), medications (especially diuretics, antiepileptics, and protease inhibitors), hypertriglyceridemia, hypercalcemia, congenital anatomic or genetic conditions (eg, pancreas divisum or cystic fibrosis transmembrane conductance regulator mutation), mumps, pancreatic neoplasm, and trauma or hypoperfusion. In 10% to 15% of cases a cause is not identified. The overall mortality is 2% to 4%.[31,32]

Pathophysiology

The pathophysiology of acute pancreatitis is poorly understood. The most common causes of acute pancreatitis can generally be broken down into mechanical (gallstones, ERCP) or systemic (alcohol, medications, hypercalcemia, hypertriglyceridemia). There are 2 suggested mechanisms whereby the mechanical causes result in acute pancreatitis: obstruction of the ampulla, or bile reflux into the pancreatic ductal system. How various systemic agents trigger acute pancreatitis is even less clear.

Most investigators agree that, whatever the inciting mechanism, acute pancreatitis result from activation of trypsin within the pancreatic acinar cells. The pancreas has mechanisms for preventing intracellular trypsin activation and counteracting low levels of activation, but when these mechanisms are overwhelmed, pancreatic autodigestion ensues, which can progress beyond the gland itself and into the surrounding peripancreatic tissues. This local injury can in turn activate a variety of systemic inflammatory mediators (complement, interleukins, phospholipase A2) that may be responsible for the systemic effects seen in severe acute pancreatitis.[32]

Diagnosis, Classification, and Severity

The diagnosis of acute pancreatitis is based on the identification of 2 of the following 3 criteria: (1) clinical: central upper abdominal pain, often with associated nausea and vomiting, and sometimes radiating to the back, (2) laboratory: serum amylase or lipase greater than 3 times the upper limit of normal, (3) radiographic: imaging (usually CT or magnetic resonance imaging [MRI]) characteristic of acute pancreatitis. Imaging is rarely required to make the diagnosis of acute pancreatitis, which can usually be made on the basis of clinical and biochemical parameters alone. Rather, imaging should be used acutely only when the diagnosis is unclear, and is typically more valuable later in the course of disease to better define local complications (discussed later in this article). The etiology of any episode of pancreatitis should be sought, as it may allow prevention of recurrent episodes. When there is no obvious inciting factor, such as heavy alcohol use or recent ERCP, abdominal ultrasound should be performed to evaluate for gallstones as a potential cause.

Terminology has been a frequent source of confusion in acute pancreatitis over the past 2 decades. An international working group recently presented revised definitions that will hopefully provide more uniformity. The severity definitions effectively stratify patients by morbidity and mortality (**Box 1**). Complex or pancreatitis-specific severity scoring systems (eg, Ranson, Glasgow, Balthazar, APACHE 2) do not perform better than these and need not be calculated. Overall, at least 80% of acute pancreatitis is mild, and 20% is severe or moderately severe.[33]

Initial Medical Management

Fluid resuscitation
Patients with severe or moderately severe pancreatitis often manifest systemic signs of inflammation (SIRS). Fluid resuscitation is required in the acute phase and based on the limited data available the fluid of choice is Ringer lactate.[34] The rate and total amount of

---

Box 1
Severity classification in acute pancreatitis

Mild Acute Pancreatitis

- No organ failure
- No local or systemic complications

Moderately Severe Acute Pancreatitis

- Organ failure that resolves within 48 hours and/or
- Local or systemic complication (without persistent organ failure)

Severe Acute Pancreatitis

- Persistent organ failure (>48 hours)

Adapted from Sarr MG, Banks PA, Bollen TL, et al. The new revised classification of acute pancreatitis 2012. Surg Clin North Am 2013;93(3):549–62.

fluid used during initial resuscitation can be difficult to calibrate. The consequences of under-resuscitation include end-organ damage and especially renal failure. Over-resuscitation can be complicated by pulmonary edema, respiratory failure, and abdominal compartment syndrome. The "sweet spot" between under-resuscitation and over-resuscitation is difficult to identify. We suggest initial resuscitation with Ringer lactate at 5 to 10 mL/kg/h with continuous reassessment of the end points of resuscitation. Relevant end points include clinical (eg, heart rate, blood pressure, urine output), invasive (eg, stroke volume variation), and biochemical (eg, hematocrit, lactate) parameters.

Nutrition

In mild pancreatitis, oral intake can be resumed as soon as abdominal pain and laboratory parameters are improving, often within the first 24 hours after presentation. Neither needs to be completely resolved before resuming oral intake. Oral intake can be rapidly advanced to a full solid diet. Indeed, one randomized controlled trial showed that initial oral intake can be with a full solid diet.[35,36] In patients with severe pancreatitis requiring nutritional supplementation, enteral feeding should be the primary therapy. No specific formulation or immunonutrition has been shown to improve outcomes. Nasogastric feeding is equivalent to nasojejunal feeding, and can be the first route of administration with nasojejunal feeding reserved for patients who do not tolerate nasogastric feeds. Parenteral nutrition should be used only in patients who cannot reach nutritional goals with enteral nutrition within 5 to 7 days.[37–40]

Antibiotics

Systemic antibiotics should be reserved for the treatment (not the prophylaxis) of infected pancreatic necrosis.[41] When treatment is initiated, carbepenems or a quinolone plus metronidazole comprises the best initial regimen based on evidence of effective pancreatic tissue penetration and an appropriate spectrum of antimicrobial activity.[42] Because fungal infection is not uncommon (25%), patients with persistently worsening clinical condition or with microbiologic evidence for fungal infection should be treated with antifungals. If cultures show Candida albicans, fluconazole is appropriate. Although good evidence for the optimal antifungal agents in pancreatitis is lacking, if the indication is severe sepsis we recommend using broader spectrum antifungal agents until definitive culture and sensitivities are available. There is some evidence that prophylactic selective digestive decontamination (SDD) with enteral antibiotics may be effective in reducing the rate of infected pancreatic necrosis, but this is not strong enough to make SDD a standard recommendation.

Imaging

CT is the most common imaging modality used for diagnosis of acute pancreatitis and its complications. As noted previously, CT is rarely needed to make the diagnosis of acute pancreatitis and should not be used routinely at the time of presentation but should be reserved for cases in which there is diagnostic uncertainty or clinical deterioration in spite of appropriate initial treatment.[43–45] Whenever possible, CT should be performed with oral and IV contrast. If CT is performed to assess for local complications and the severity of the pancreatitis, the optimal timing is 72 to 96 hours after presentation, as CT scans performed in the first 72 hours frequently underestimate the degree of pancreatic and peripancreatic necrosis. Even when early CT shows significant abnormalities, follow-up imaging is not recommended unless there is clinical deterioration or lack of improvement. A patient who continues to improve after an episode of acute pancreatitis, even a severe episode with documented necrosis, does not require serial imaging to monitor resolution. MRI can provide most of the same information as CT. Potential advantages include the lack of ionizing radiation and superiority in delineating liquid and solid components within peripancreatic necrosis. As noted earlier in the Diagnosis section, early ultrasonography should also be used to assess for gallstones as the source of the pancreatitis episode if no other etiology is apparent.

Intervention

Initial medical management for pancreatitis can be easily provided at most hospitals, but intervention requires a facility with a multidisciplinary team including at least surgeons, interventional radiologists, and gastroenterologists experienced in managing the disease.[46] The clearest consensus indication for intervention is infected pancreatic necrosis. Infected necrosis can be diagnosed definitively by the finding of air in an area of pancreatic necrosis on CT scanning or by Gram stain and culture of a fine-needle aspirate (FNA) of the necrosis. However, infected necrosis is a clinical diagnosis, and experienced clinicians are as accurate as invasive testing in detecting it. It is important to remember that FNA is only approximately 65% sensitive for the diagnosis of infection. Thus, patients who are clinically unwell with suspicion for infected necrosis should be treated as if they have infection, as there is no reliable means to exclude it, and the consequences of missing it are grave.

Once the diagnosis of infected necrosis is made, treatment is with the supportive care described previously. When possible, in stable patients intervention should be delayed to 28 days or more from the onset of the pancreatitis episode. This may be impossible if patients are clinically unstable. Whenever the first intervention is undertaken, a minimally invasive percutaneous or endoscopic drainage procedure should be the initial procedure as the first step in a so-called "step-up" approach.[47,48] Between 20% and 45% of patients with infected necrosis can be successfully treated with percutaneous or endoscopic drainage alone, although this may require several repeat drainage procedures. Drains should be placed taking into account the planned strategies for subsequent stages of the step-up approach. When possible, this may involve placing at least one drain into the area of infected necrosis via a retroperitoneal route to allow for video-assisted retroperitoneal debridement (VARD) along the drain tract (Fig. 5). VARD involves a small subcostal flank incision, dissection along the drain tract into the necrosis cavity, and blunt debridement of the necrotic and infected fluid and tissue. Long retractors are used to expose the tract and cavity and a standard laparoscope is used to improve visualization of the cavity, although there is no insufflation.[49] For patients with necrosis anatomically amenable to such a "step-up" approach, short-term benefits include the ability to avoid any surgery in a significant subset of the population and less new-onset organ failure. Long-term benefits include reduced incidence of diabetes mellitus and incisional hernia. For patients debrided entirely via an endoscopic route, there also may be a mortality advantage compared with open surgery without any preoperative drainage procedure.[50]

Due to the anatomy of their necrosis, some patients with infected pancreatic necrosis will not be amenable to endoscopic or retroperitoneal debridement, in which case laparotomy or less commonly laparoscopy may be used for transperitoneal debridement. Additionally, it must be noted that although minimally invasive drainage as a first step likely confers significant advantages, when surgery is subsequently required, the evidence is less compelling that any one surgical approach is superior to others. The general principles of delay until 4 weeks after the onset of disease and preoperative drainage of some form should still be applied whatever the approach. Transabdominal debridement should involve removal of all or nearly all infected or necrotic pancreatic and peripancreatic tissue with closed suction drainage of the

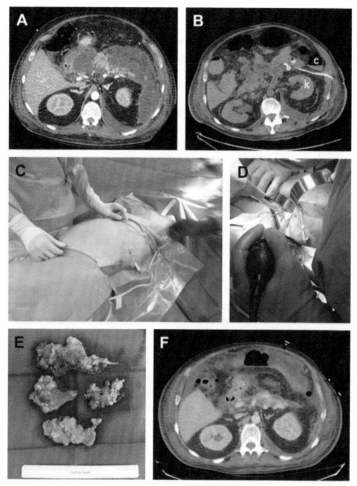

Fig. 5. Video-assisted retroperitoneal pancreatic debridement (VARD). (*A*) CT scan showing walled off pancreatic necrosis amenable to retroperitoneal access. (*B*) Percutaneous drain placed via a retroperitoneal route to guide VARD. C, colon; K, kidney. (*C*) Positioning in the operating room with right side elevated and percutaneous drain prepped into the operative field. (*D*) Dissecting along the percutaneous drain tract into the necrosis cavity. (*E*) Necrotic pancreatic tissue removed by VARD. The ruler is 15 cm long. (*F*) Postoperative CT scan showing resolution of the necrosis cavity.

necrotic cavity. The use of different incisions (midline vs subcostal), approaches to the pancreas (transmesocolic, through the gastrocolic omentum, or retroperitoneal), and drainage (closed packing, closed suction alone, continuous lavage) are at the discretion of the surgeon and acceptable results can be obtained with variable techniques.[51]

Intervention is less often needed for sterile pancreatic necrosis. The most common indication is gastric outlet obstruction. Intervention can often be delayed longer, as this complication will often resolve with time. If patients with presumed sterile necrosis remain persistently unwell, the possibility of occult infection must be considered. Intervention can include surgical debridement or bypass.

Other complications that may prompt intervention in the acute setting include abdominal compartment syndrome (ACS), hemorrhage of a visceral artery (usually splenic artery) pseudoaneurysm, and bowel perforation or fistula. When these complications arise in the acute setting they should, as a rule, be treated by the least invasive methods possible. For ACS, medical treatment should include volume removal (via diuresis or ultrafiltration), and neuromuscular blockade. If there is persistent ACS and significant ascites, percutaneous drainage may be beneficial, and is currently under investigation in a randomized trial.[52] Definitive treatment is decompressive laparotomy.[53] When this is necessary early in the course of disease, the lesser sac should not be entered and pancreatic debridement should be avoided. Bleeding from a visceral artery pseudoaneurysm should be controlled endovascularly by angioembolization whenever possible, as direct surgical control in a region of active or recent pancreatitis is extremely difficult.[54] Intestinal perforation is similarly difficult to manage. Contained perforations or controlled fistulas may be manageable with drainage or diversion. When there is bowel ischemia or uncontrolled enteric spillage, exploratory laparotomy with resection will likely be necessary.

Late Complications

Pancreatic fistulas and pseudocysts result from disruption of the pancreatic duct due to destruction of the surrounding parenchyma. Fistulas may result from severe pancreatitis or as a complication of pancreatic debridement, after which they are common. One advantage of endoscopic transluminal debridement may be that such leaks from the pancreatic duct drain internally, rather than forming external fistulas. Whatever the cause, when the fistula is controlled with percutaneous drains, it will usually close, although it may require many weeks to months. Pancreatic duct stenting, octreotide administration, and restriction of enteral nutrition have all been advocated to aid in fistula closure, but are not routinely helpful. In the special situation of a disconnected distal pancreatic remnant in which a segment of the gland has been completely separated from any route of drainage into the gastrointestinal tract, spontaneous closure is very rare. Such patients may be treated either endoscopically by transluminal stenting to attempt to convert the external fistula into a controlled internal fistula, or may be treated surgically by either roux-en-Y jejunostomy to the distal pancreatic remnant or resection of the disconnected distal segment.

Pseudocysts form when the ductal disruption is walled off by the body into an organized collection of pancreatic juice encased by reactive inflammatory tissue, a process that occurs 4 weeks or more after damage to the pancreatic duct. Asymptomatic pseudocysts do not require intervention. The most common symptoms are early satiety and abdominal pain. Pseudocysts may also cause true gastric outlet obstruction, become infected, or lead to pseudoaneurysm formation. Internal drainage is the treatment of choice for pseudocysts requiring intervention. For pseudocysts closely apposed to the stomach or duodenum, endoscopic pseudocyst-gastrostomy or duodenostomy is the treatment of choice. For very large or endoscopically inaccessible pseudocysts, surgical cyst gastrostomy or roux-en-Y cyst jejunostomy are necessary.[55]

Vascular complications of pancreatitis include arterial pseudoaneurysm and venous thrombosis. These most commonly involve the splenic vessels, but in pancreatitis primarily affecting the head, pseudoaneurysms of the pancreaticoduodenal or gastroduodenal arteries may occur along with thrombosis of the superior mesenteric or portal veins. Pseuodaneurysms result from the action of pancreatic enzymes on the arterial wall. They may be identified incidentally on contrast-enhanced CT or can present with catastrophic hemorrhage. We recommend intervening even on asymptomatic pseudoaneurysms in most cases, as there is no reliable way to predict hemorrhage. As noted previously, whether addressed electively or emergently they are best treated with angioembolization.[54] Splenic vein thrombosis due to pancreatitis can usually be observed. We occasionally anticoagulate if clot extends into the main portal vein. Even without anticoagulation, the thrombus can resolve. If it does not, the most common late complication is gastric varices. If these result in gastrointestinal bleeding, they can be eliminated by splenectomy.[56]

Efforts should be made to prevent recurrence after an episode of pancreatitis by cessation of ethanol abuse for alcoholic pancreatitis, treatment of the underlying condition in hypercalcemia and hypertriglyceridemia, and cessation of any offending medications in cases of medication-induced pancreatitis. In patients with gallstone pancreatitis, cholecystectomy during the same hospitalization is recommended for mild cases. In pancreatitis with peripancreatic fluid collections, cholecystectomy should be delayed for 6 weeks. In especially poor operative candidates, ERCP with sphincterotomy reduces the risk of recurrent gallstone pancreatitis and can be considered as an alternative to cholecystectomy.

DIVERTICULITIS

Key points

- Colonoscopy should be performed after an episode of diverticulitis unless the patient has had a recent one.
- Diverticular abscess should be treated with percutaneous drainage and antibiotics. Elective laparoscopic colectomy after resolution should usually be undertaken.
- Emergency sigmoid colectomy is rarely required for acute diverticulitis.
- When emergency sigmoid colectomy is required, primary anastomosis with or without diverting ileostomy should be strongly considered.
- The utility and role of laparoscopic lavage has yet to be determined.

The management of sigmoid diverticulitis in all its manifestations has changed considerably in recent years. Indications for elective or emergency surgery, choices of surgical approach, and methods for preventing recurrence are all evolving. This review discusses these issues with a focus on the acute management of complicated diverticulitis.

Epidemiology and Etiology

Diverticulitis is the third most common cause of hospitalization due to gastrointestinal disease in the United States, with an estimated 219,000 visits in 2009, and the incidence is increasing.[30,57] The prevalence of diverticulosis is age dependent and in the United States is approximately 20% by age 40, rising to 60% by age 60. Suggested risk factors for diverticulosis include low dietary fiber intake, obesity, and lack of physical activity. In a recent longitudinal study of patients with incidentally identified diverticulosis, the subsequent risk of developing diverticulitis was approximately 4.3% over 11 years of follow-up.[58] Seasonal and regional variations in hospital admissions for diverticulitis have been noted in the United States, although what drives these variations is unclear. A minority of episodes of diverticulitis require hospital admission, but hospitalized patients younger than 45 are more likely to be men, whereas women comprise most patients hospitalized in those older than 54.[57] The overall incidence of diverticulitis continues to increase with increasing age. After a first episode of diverticulitis, 20% to 40% of patients develop recurrent diverticulitis, with a similar percentage of those patients going on to develop a third episode.[59] Most patients with complicated diverticular disease (perforation, abscess, fistula, or stricture) have never had prior episodes of acute diverticulitis.[60]

Pathophysiology

The pathophysiology of colonic diverticula formation is incompletely understood. Colonic diverticula are pseudodiverticula composed of mucosal and submucosal layers only. The colon may be anatomically predisposed to formation of these diverticulae because the muscular layers are not circumferential and because of weakness at the site of entrance of the vasa recta. At the microscopic level, collagen cross-linking increases with age and increased elastin deposition has been noted in the colon of patients with diverticulosis. These processes may result in a highly contractile and less distensible colon, which is predisposed to segmentation, the phenomenon when adjacent haustra simultaneously contract creating a short closed segment of colon with very high intraluminal pressure. Low-fiber diets are associated with diverticula formation, although the pathophysiologic link is not completely clear. Less stool bulk may predispose to segmentation and higher intraluminal pressures. Other environmental or genetic predispositions are suggested by the observation that right-sided diverticulosis and diverticulitis is significantly more common in Asia than in Western countries, and by the high prevalence of diverticulosis in patients with certain connective tissue disorders, such as Ehlers-Danlos syndrome. Thus anatomic factors probably interact with functional and environmental factors to form diverticulae.[61,62] Diverticulitis results from acute inflammation of a diverticulum. When this leads to perforation, complicated disease ensues. The factors that initiate inflammation and lead to micro or gross perforation are poorly understood. Diverticular obstruction, colonic stasis, changes in the local bacterial biome, and local ischemia have all been implicated.

Diagnosis, Classification, and Severity

Evaluation of a patient with suspected diverticulitis should include a history focused on localizing pain, eliciting evidence of possible prior episodes, and identifying clinical evidence of complicated disease (obstructive symptoms, pneumaturia, fecaluria, or vaginal discharge). Pain is usually in the lower abdomen and the differential diagnosis includes appendicitis, infectious or ischemic colitis, inflammatory bowel disease, nephrolithiasis, and gynecologic pathology. The abdominal examination usually reveals focal left lower quadrant or suprapubic tenderness. The diagnosis can be made without laboratory testing or radiologic imaging in clinically mild cases, especially in patients with a history of the disease. In patients never previously diagnosed, or those who appear systemically ill, laboratory evaluation should include a complete blood count and urinalysis. CT scanning with oral and IV contrast is by far the most useful diagnostic modality in suspected acute diverticulitis, as it is both sensitive and specific, can evaluate the other diagnostic possibilities, and can identify complications, such as abscess, fistula, or obstruction. CT cannot, however, definitively differentiate between diverticulitis and colonic adenocarcinoma. Because as many as 3% to 5% of cases of clinically diagnosed diverticulitis may turn out to be adenocarcinoma, colonoscopy or other appropriate colorectal cancer screening should be performed after resolution of the acute episode unless patients have had a recent screening evaluation and have a known diagnosis of recurrent diverticulitis.

Surgeons are usually involved in the care of patients with acute diverticulitis when they manifest systemic symptoms, fail to improve with medical therapy, or develop complicated disease. Complicated disease refers to diverticulitis associated with abscess, fistula, perforation, stricture, or obstruction. For cases of perforation, the Hinchey classification is the most commonly used schema (**Box 2**).

Specific Diverticulitis Entities and Their Management

Uncomplicated diverticulitis is typically treated with 7 to 14 days of antibiotics and bowel rest until symptoms improve, at which point the diet is gradually reintroduced starting with liquids. The need for antibiotics in the treatment of acute uncomplicated diverticulitis has recently been challenged by a multicenter randomized controlled trial that showed no difference in hospital stay, the development of complications, or recurrence rates between patients randomized to receive antibiotics and those randomized not to receive them. Only 3% of patients in the no-antibiotic arm crossed over to the antibiotic arm due to worsening pain or fever.[63] Although the necessity of antibiotics in mild diverticulitis will likely continue to be investigated, they are still considered standard in mild disease and are a mainstay of treatment in complicated disease. Antibiotic regimens should cover enteric gram-negative organisms and anaerobes. Ciprofloxacin and metronidazole is the most common regimen; alternatives include a beta-lactam/beta-lactamase combination (amoxicillin/clavulanic acid or piperacillin/tazobactam), substitution of clindamycin for metronidazole, and moxifloxacin or a carbapenem as monotherapy.[7,64] Patients with systemic inflammatory response syndrome or organ failure due to complicated diverticulitis should be resuscitated appropriately, in an intensive care unit if necessary. Even in the setting of free perforation requiring surgery, most septic patients will benefit from at least a brief period of preoperative resuscitation.

The most common complication of diverticulitis is abscess, which is typically diagnosed on CT, and the mainstay of therapy, is percutaneous radiologically guided drainage. The Hinchey classification distinguishes between localized pericolonic abscess and pelvic abscesses. Many Hinchey I and small Hinchey II abscesses can be treated with antibiotics alone. The American Society of Colon and Rectal Surgeons recommends antibiotic therapy alone for abscesses smaller than 2 cm. A retrospective study demonstrated 100% success in the acute treatment of diverticular abscesses smaller than 3 cm, and other studies have called into question the necessity of draining intermediate-sized abscesses (3–5 cm).[65,66] The question of how large an abscess can be before it requires percutaneous drainage is in evolution. A combined evaluation of the patient's clinical condition and the radiographic characteristics of the abscess is the most rational approach to intermediate-sized abscesses at this time. A medium-sized abscess (eg, 4 cm) that is difficult or

---

Box 2
Hinchey classification for perforated diverticulitis

Stage I: pericolic or mesenteric abscess

Stage II: walled off pelvic abscess

Stage III: generalized purulent peritonitis

Stage IV: generalized fecal peritonitis

Adapted from Hinchey EJ, Schaal PG, Richards GK. Treatment of perforated diverticular disease of the colon. Adv Surg 1978;12:85.

dangerous to access percutaneously in a patient who is clinically well should probably be treated initially with antibiotics alone, whereas a similar-sized abscess that is easily accessible in a patient with severe pain or persistent fever should be drained. In patients initially managed with antibiotics alone, drainage should be undertaken if technically feasible in the absence of clinical improvement. The success rate with percutaneous drainage is in the range of 60% to 85%. Drains are typically removed when imaging shows resolution of the abscess cavity and output is low (<10–20 mL/24 hours). The surgical options for failed nonoperative management are discussed as follows.

Diverticular stricture is the second most common cause of large bowel obstruction in the United States. Even when a benign etiology is strongly suggested, it is difficult to definitively rule out malignancy, and so resection is usually required to prevent recurrent obstruction and rule out or treat possible malignancy. Most obstructions due to diverticulitis are incomplete and result from inflammation or edema superimposed on a chronic stricture during an acute flare of diverticulitis. With treatment, the acute obstruction may resolve, allowing decompression and elective single-stage resection. When obstruction is high grade, the options are immediate resection or performance of a procedure to temporarily relieve the obstruction. We favor resection with primary anastomosis whenever possible. On table lavage of the proximal colon has not been shown to have any advantage over manual decompression of the proximal colon; therefore, we do not routinely perform or recommend it.[67] Whether a proximal diverting loop ileostomy is necessary when resection and anastomosis is performed remains a matter of debate. Reports indicate that anastomosis without proximal diversion can be performed safely, but it has not been studied in a controlled fashion and for now can be left to individual surgeon judgment.[68] Patients with metabolic derangement, severe malnutrition, or other reasons not to undergo immediate resection may benefit from a temporizing procedure to relieve the obstruction. Colonic stents have an excellent track record for relief of malignant large bowel obstruction, but are associated with a much higher complication rate when used for diverticular stricture and should be used only very selectively if at all.[69] For the rare patients who are acutely ill from large bowel obstruction or in imminent danger of cecal perforation (cecum >10 cm), a temporary transverse loop colostomy remains a good option; it can be safely performed quickly, even under local anesthesia if needed due to hemodynamic instability, and relieves the obstruction. It can be closed at the time of subsequent resection and primary anastomosis. As mentioned previously, this is rarely necessary and resection with primary anastomosis is usually preferred.

Free perforation is generally associated with diffuse peritonitis on abdominal examination, widespread uncontained pneumoperitoneum and free fluid on CT scan, and signs of severe systemic infection. It is important to note that pneumoperitoneum alone, even large-volume pneumoperitoneum, is not a reliable sign of ongoing free perforation nor is it an indication for surgery. Diverticular perforations will often seal, and patients with pneumoperitoneum who do not otherwise clinically or radiographically manifest ongoing fecal spillage may still be managed nonoperatively.[70] Patients with ongoing free perforation require broad-spectrum antibiotics and fluid resuscitation, as noted previously, but also require surgical intervention. Surgical options include sigmoid colectomy with end colostomy (Hartmann procedure), sigmoid colectomy with primary colorectal anastomosis with or without diverting loop ileostomy, and laparoscopic lavage with primary closure of the perforation. The Hartmann procedure has been less frequently used in recent years, as awareness of the morbidity of colostomy reversal has increased. In general, it should be used mostly in patients for whom a permanent end colostomy would be acceptable, such as patients with dementia or incontinence, in whom it may actually be a boon. Otherwise, primary anastomosis with diverting loop ileostomy appears to be as safe in the short term, and to be accompanied by much higher rates of stoma closure, a lower rate of serious complications, shorter hospital stay, and lower costs.[71]

The role of laparoscopic lavage in the management of diverticular perforations is unclear. Numerous single-center series report good outcomes. The primary problem with these is the lack of comparative data. Many patients with Hinchey III for whom the procedure is most ardently advocated are likely to improve with medical management alone. Case series beg the question: was any surgery needed at all? There is no definitive data indicating that laparoscopic lavage adds anything to a combination of antibiotic treatment and percutaneous radiologically guided drainage of localized collections. Advocates of the technique differ on whether it is appropriate in patients with Hinchey IV disease, whether ongoing perforation with leakage should be actively sought either preoperatively or intraoperatively, and whether a finding of perforation or stool spillage constitutes a reason to convert to a sigmoid resection or whether a simple laparoscopic repair as part of the lavage procedure is appropriate. Defining the appropriate role for this technique is one of the larger unanswered questions in the current acute surgical management of complicated diverticulitis and would benefit greatly from a randomized trial.[72]

Prevention of Recurrence

We typically recommend colonoscopy 6 weeks after a first episode of acute diverticulitis and in patients who are otherwise due for colorectal cancer screening. In one large series of 319 patients, 89% of patients had the diagnosis of diverticulitis confirmed, and 26% of these had adenomatous polyps identified. Nine patients (2.8%) had an unsuspected colorectal cancer identified.[73] If the episode of diverticulitis is confirmed, patients are often anxious to know what they can do to prevent recurrences. Advice on this topic has been clouded by decades of myth surrounding dietary modifications. Although the ideal diet to prevent recurrent diverticulitis is not known, the avoidance of seeds and nuts, which have been baselessly demonized for decades, is not necessary. Debate remains over whether high-fiber diets can prevent recurrent symptoms, and whether low-residue diets improve symptoms in the setting of an acute flair. This debate can still rage largely unchecked by evidence. High-fiber diets are supported by some evidence, are unlikely to cause harm, and are still recommended in a number of professional society guidelines for prevention of recurrent diverticulitis; we recommend them, but without much enthusiasm.[74] Medical therapy, including intermittent luminal antibiotics, probiotics, and 5-aminosalicylic acid, has been investigated for prevention of recurrent diverticulitis. These remain options for patients with multiply recurrent disease who are poor candidates for or decline surgery (discussed later), but all these interventions require further investigation before they can be routinely recommended. The 5-aminosalicylic acid therapy has the best support in the form of a randomized controlled trial.[75,76]

Guidelines for elective sigmoid resection to prevent recurrent diverticulitis have evolved considerably in the past decade, but are not governed by clear evidence and still recommend making decisions on a case-by-case basis considering the severity of the episode(s) and the medical condition and age of the patient. For patients suffering an episode of complicated diverticulitis requiring percutaneous abscess drainage, the incidence of recurrent severe sepsis may be as high as 41%, and thus interval sigmoid colectomy should usually be planned.[77] This constitutes one of the clearer indications for elective sigmoid resection, although even in this setting nonoperative management can be considered in elderly or poor-risk patients, in whom recurrence is common, but can typically be managed nonoperatively with minimal morbidity.[78] The number of uncomplicated episodes that should prompt resection is less clear, as is the impact that age should have on decision making. Approximately one-third of patients will suffer recurrence after a single episode of uncomplicated acute diverticulitis, and another third of those develop a third episode. If the first episode was uncomplicated, the subsequent episodes usually are, thus early surgery in this setting is unlikely to prevent complicated and morbid episodes of diverticulitis. We rarely offer colectomy if there have been fewer than 3 episodes. Modifying considerations may include the presence of immunosuppression, chronic renal failure, or collagen vascular disease, all of which confer a significantly increased risk of subsequently developing complicated disease, or the presence of persistent symptoms between acute episodes. We recommend laparoscopic colectomy as the preferred method of resection based on an overall lower morbidity rate in experienced hands.[79]

CLOSTRIDIUM DIFFICILE COLITIS

Key points

- Oral vancomycin is standard treatment for moderate to severe Clostridium difficile infection (CDI), and can be supplemented with intravenous metronidazole and vancomycin enemas in severe cases.
- Fidaxomicin reduces recurrent CDI compared with standard therapy.
- Patients developing new or worsening organ failure on appropriate medical therapy need surgery.
- Surgical options include subtotal colectomy with end ileostomy, or loop ileostomy with antegrade colonic lavage.
- Fidaxomicin, tapered intermittent vancomycin, and fecal bacteriotherapy are options for recalcitrant recurrent CDI.

Clostridium difficile infection (CDI) is one of the most common hospital-acquired infections, and is a frequent cause of morbidity and mortality among hospitalized patients. C difficile colonizes the intestinal tract after the normal gut flora has been altered by antibiotic therapy. Most CDI is relatively mild, but a minority of patients (3%–12%) can progress to severe disease resulting in systemic toxicity and shock. This subset is the primary concern of the acute care surgeon.

Epidemiology and Etiology

CDI afflicts up to 10% of all hospitalized patients and 20% of such patients receiving antibiotics.[80] A study using the Nationwide Inpatient Sample showed a 109% increase in incidence of C difficile infections between 1993 and 2003.[80] More recent national data showed that the rate of C difficile hospitalizations per 1000 nonmaternal, adult discharges increased from about 5.6 in 2001 to 12.8 in 2012, with annual costs in the United States estimated in the billions of dollars.[81,82] Two percent to 8% of patients with CDI will develop fulminant disease, defined as CDI with significant systemic toxic effects and shock, resulting in the need for intensive care unit (ICU) admission, colectomy, or death.[80,83,84] Mortality rates for fulminant CDI range between 13.8% and 80.0%.[83,84] These increases in the incidence, prevalence, severity, and recurrence rates of CDI have been closely linked to the development of the hypervirulent NAP1/BI/027 strain.[85]

Risk factors for CDI include antibiotic exposure, institutionalization (including hospitalization and nursing home residence), advanced age, severe illness, and gastric acid suppression (especially with proton pump inhibitors). The antibiotics most commonly associated with CDI are flouroquinolones, although a very wide array of antibiotics have been implicated and the disease can even occur in the absence of antibiotic exposure.[85,86]

Pathophysiology

C difficile is an anaerobic gram-positive, spore-forming, toxin-producing bacillus. Outside the colon, it survives in spore form and is highly resistant to heat, acid, and antibiotics. This feature is closely linked to its nosocomial spread. Currently, full-contact precautions (gown and gloves) as well as hand washing with soap and water in addition to use of an alcohol-based hand rub (ABHR) are recommended for health care providers contacting patients with *C difficile*. ABHRs alone are inadequate to eradicate spores. Similarly, special precautions are required for cleaning of the health care environment (usually sodium hypochlorite solutions) and potential fomites (such as stethoscopes) which require sporicidal wipes.[87] On reaching the colon, spores convert to the vegetative, toxin-producing forms that result in clinical infection and are susceptible to antimicrobial agents. The vegetative form of *C difficile* releases 2 exotoxins that mediate colitis and diarrhea: toxin A ("enterotoxin") and toxin B ("cytotoxin"). These toxins cause mucosal cell death, resulting in the classic pseudomembranes seen on endoscopy (**Fig. 6**), disrupting the gut barrier, and leading in severe cases to a toxic megacolon picture. Stool toxin levels correlate with disease severity, whereas host antitoxin antibodies are inversely correlated with infection incidence, severity, and recurrence.

Diagnosis, Classification, and Severity

Watery diarrhea is the clinical hallmark of CDI, although clinical manifestations of disease can range from none (asymptomatic carrier status) to fulminant septic shock. CDI

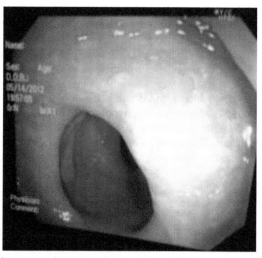

Fig. 6. Pseudomembranous colitis in a patient with *C difficile* infection. Note the edematous mucosa and exudative pseudomembranes.

should be suspected in any hospitalized patient with diarrhea and appropriate testing should be performed to confirm the diagnosis (see later in this article). As awareness of the prevalence of CDI has increased in recent years, infection is probably promptly suspected and diagnosed in most cases with diarrhea. Surgeons caring for hospitalized inpatients will frequently encounter other presentations in which diarrhea is absent, however. These situations can constitute more of a diagnostic challenge. Unexplained leukocytosis, even in the absence of diarrhea should raise suspicion for CDI. Pancolitis seen on imaging performed for other symptoms (such as abdominal pain, nausea, vomiting, or fever) is also an occasional first indicator of colitis and CDI.

When CDI is suspected, the diagnosis should be confirmed by laboratory studies or endoscopy. Laboratory studies performed on stool form the foundation of diagnosis. Most clinical laboratories rely on enzyme immunoassay (EIA) toxin testing due to a combination of rapid turnaround time, low cost, and decent sensitivity and specificity. Because a certain quantity of toxin (100–1000 pg) must be present to allow detection, sensitivity may be as low as 75%, however. This is minimally improved by sending samples on consecutive days, which unearths a new positive test less than 3% of the time. We consider polymerase chain reaction (PCR), which has sensitivities and specificities in the 93% to 97% range, as the best single stool test for CDI. In clinical microbiology laboratories, both PCR and EIA are often used as part of a multistep diagnostic algorithm because of their cost and lack of sensitivity respectively. Clinicians should understand the testing algorithm used at their institution and its performance characteristics.[88]

Colonoscopy or sigmoidoscopy is unnecessary when a patient has diarrhea and a positive stool sample, but may be diagnostically useful in certain situations. These include when suspicion for CDI remains high despite negative laboratory tests, when an immediate diagnosis is necessary, and when the diagnosis is suspected but due to ileus, no stool is available for diagnostic testing. Pseudomembranes are specific for CDI in the proper clinical setting and are a marker for severe disease. The chief drawback to endoscopy is the risk of perforation, which likely increases with the severity of colonic inflammation, although we have never experienced this. In patients with advanced colitis, abdominal CT shows marked colonic thickening in a pancolonic distribution, although *C difficile* colitis is not distinguishable radiographically from other forms of infectious colitis.

There are no established criteria for differentiating "mild to moderate" from "severe" CDI. Different investigators have used slightly different criteria in studies. The distinction is ultimately clinical and based on an assessment of colonic disease severity and systemic effects. Criteria to be considered include the following: number of bowel movements (>10–12, severe); presence of abdominal pain or tenderness, leukocytosis, or leukopenia (white blood cell count >15–20,000 or <4000, severe); fever; elevated serum lactate (>2.2); tachycardia; hypotension or need for vasopressors; respiratory failure; age (>60–70); pseudomembranes on endoscopy, or extensive colonic wall thickening on CT scan. Any patient requiring admission to an ICU for treatment of CDI should be considered to have severe disease and treated accordingly.

Initial Medical Management

A combined algorithm for medical and surgical management used since 2007 as a guideline in the Division of Trauma, Emergency Surgery, and Critical Care at the Massachusetts General Hospital is provided in **Fig. 7**. The criteria used to help determine the need for surgery were chosen because they were highly associated with mortality in a retrospective study from our institution.[83] The first steps in treatment of CDI are cessation of the inciting antibiotic as soon as possible, and standard supportive

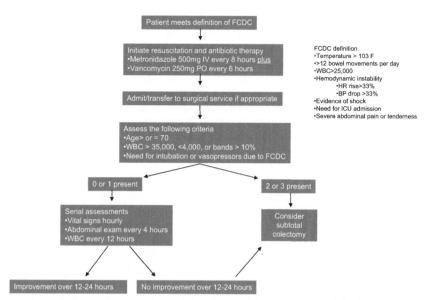

Fig. 7. Suggested algorithm for determining the need for surgery in *C difficile* colitis. *Abbreviations*: FCDC, fulminant *C difficile* colitics; ICU, intensive care unit; IV, intravenous; PO, by mouth; WBC, white blood cell count.

therapy, such as intravascular volume restoration, and correction of electrolyte abnormalities. Enteral feeding should be used whenever possible. Patients with severe disease should be serially examined and moved to monitored settings (ICU or observation unit) as appropriate based on their physiology.

Antibiotics targeted at *C difficile* form the mainstay of medical management. For nonsevere disease, oral metronidazole is the first line agent of choice. The recommended dosage and duration of therapy for nonsevere disease is 500 mg 3 times per day for 10 to 14 days or at least 7 days beyond the cessation of any inciting antibiotics. Oral vancomycin is a standard alternative. Vancomycin 125 mg orally 4 times per day for the same duration is an alternative dose for nonsevere disease. For severe disease, oral vancomycin is first-line therapy. Dosing can be anywhere from 125 mg to 500 mg 4 times per day. There is some evidence that higher colonic vancomycin levels are achieved at higher doses, but no clear evidence of clinical benefit. Severely ill patients with CDI often have ileus with delayed transit of oral vancomycin into the colon. For this reason, we routinely use IV metronidazole (500 mg every 6–8 hours) in conjunction with oral vancomycin when initiating antibiotic therapy in severe CDI. If patients do not show improvement with this regimen, intracolonic vancomycin is an additional option. The ideal method of administration has not been carefully defined, but 500 mg given in 100 mL normal saline every 6 hours as a retention enema is a standard regimen. Fidaxomicin is a relatively new macrocyclic antibiotic with bactericidal activity against *C difficile* (in contrast to vancomycin and metronidazole, which are bacteristatic). It has equal short-term efficacy to oral vancomycin, but results in less recurrent CDI.[89] Its exact role in the antibiotic armamentarium has yet to be defined, but if available, it is a reasonable addition to the standard regimen in the absence of clinical improvement.

Recurrent CDI is a common problem, affecting approximately 25% of patients initially treated successfully. Some authorities recommend treating first recurrences with the same antibiotic used to treat the index infection. This has the advantage of simplicity, but is associated with a subsequent recurrence rate of approximately 50%.[90] Fidaxomicin has a lower rate of subsequent recurrences when used to treat a first recurrence.[91] For first recurrences that are moderate to severe or for second recurrences, an intermittent tapered vancomycin (125 mg twice daily for 7 days, then once daily for 7 days, then every other day for 7 days, then every third day for 2 weeks) is more effective than standard antimicrobial regimens at preventing subsequent recurrences.[92] Fecal bacteriotherapy in which donor stool is prepared and infused into the gastrointestinal tract of patients with recurrent CDI is also effective in reducing subsequent recurrences, although is not currently widely available.[93]

Surgery

Surgery is necessary for medically refractory CDI that progresses to the systemic inflammatory response syndrome causing multiorgan failure, toxic megacolon, and perforation or impending perforation. The 2 main questions confronting the surgeon are (1) when to operate, and (2) what operation to perform. The timing of surgery in severe *C difficile* colitis remains a difficult clinical judgment. Generally, we favor early surgery in patients with signs of organ failure. A significant number of patients who are hypotensive on initial presentation because of severe volume depletion from diarrhea and who have not yet been treated medically will respond quickly to volume restoration and antibiotic therapy. This should be attempted with careful observation. Those who do not respond, and any patients developing respiratory failure, renal failure, or refractory hypotension should undergo prompt surgery before a prolonged period of organ failure has resulted in an unrecoverable situation. Patients developing new organ failure due to CDI while on appropriate medical therapy should undergo surgery promptly, as there is no other therapy available that can reasonably be expected to turn the tide. Surgery offers the best chance of cure when performed before severe, prolonged, multisystem failure has developed.[83]

Subtotal colectomy (resection of the colon from the ileocecal valve to the rectum at the peritoneal reflection) is the appropriate surgical intervention for severe CDI mandating surgery. Given the indications for surgery (shock, organ failure) anastomosis should not be performed, instead leaving an end ileostomy and a rectal stump. At exploration, the colon is usually extremely boggy and dilated. If surgery is performed promptly, as recommended previously, frank necrosis or perforation is unusual. There is no role for segmental colonic resection in CDI; the infection is a pancolonic process and segmental resection will not adequately relieve the systemic toxin burden. Partial colonic resection has been associated with high mortality rates.[94] After subtotal colectomy, we usually continue IV metronidazole for 7 days to treat residual disease in the rectum. If there is evidence of ongoing proctitis, then vancomycin enemas as described previously are administered into the rectal stump. After resolution of the acute illness, ileorectal anastomosis can be performed to restore gastrointestinal continuity, although given the numerous comorbidities and advanced age of many patients requiring surgery, this is performed in only a minority of patients.

One intriguing approach to the surgical treatment of medically refractory CDI is ileostomy with colonic lavage. In this technique, a loop ileostomy is created in the terminal ileum, either laparoscopically, or using an open technique. Intraoperative antegrade colonic lavage is then performed with polyethylene glycol via a catheter introduced into the distal limb of the ileostomy. Postoperatively, the catheter is left in place, and antegrade enteral vancomycin is administered. In the experience reported to date, this approach is effective in treating colitis and preserving the colon more than 90% of the time with an acceptable mortality (21%) and a high rate of ileostomy reversal.[95] Despite exciting early results, this technique has not been directly compared with subtotal colectomy in any organized trial and we cannot yet recommend it as standard therapy, although it holds promise for the future. We currently perform it only very selectively outside of an ongoing randomized trial.

Nonstandard Agents: Monoclonal Antibodies, Anion-Binding Resins, Fecal Bacteriotherapy, Intravenous Immunoglobulin

Therapies aimed at the C difficile toxin itself have the theoretical advantage of not further disturbing the colonic flora while attenuating the systemic inflammatory response. Monoclonal antibodies directed at toxins A and B have been shown to reduce recurrence compared with vancomycin in a randomized controlled trial, but are not widely clinically available.[96] Anion-binding resins, such as colestipol, cholestyramine, and tolevamer, have not been shown to be as effective as standard antibiotics in treating C difficile colitis, but may have an adjunctive role, particularly for treating recurrent C difficile colitis. They should be used carefully, as they may also bind enteral vancomycin, thus reducing efficacy, and dosing regimens need to be carefully coordinated. Intravenous immunoglobulin contains C difficile antitoxin, and case reports describe benefit in refractory C difficile infection. No benefit has been shown in case-controlled studies and no trials have been done. We do not recommend its use.

Since a disruption of normal colonic flora underlies the pathophysiology of C difficile infection, efforts to therapeutically alter colonic flora have been made. Probiotic therapy with live bacterial cultures has been disappointing in either preventing or eliminating CDI. Fecal bacteriotherapy, or "stool transplantation" as it is sometime colloquially termed, was discussed previously, and has been shown to be effective for severe and recurrent CDI, although the infrastructure to safely perform this technique is not widely available.

REFERENCES

1. Addiss DG, Shaffer N, Fowler BS, et al. The epidemiology of appendicitis and appendectomy in the United States. Am J Epidemiol 1990;132:910–25.
2. Prystowsky JB, Pugh CM, Nagle AP. Current problems in surgery: appendicitis. Curr Probl Surg 2005;42:688–742.
3. Andersen RE. Meta-analysis of the clinical and laboratory of diagnosis of appendicitis. Br J Surg 2004;91:28–37.
4. Flum DR, Koepsell T. The clinical and economic correlates of misdiagnosed appendicitis: nationwide analysis. Arch Surg 2002;137:799–804.
5. Alvarado A. A practical score for the early diagnosis of acute appendicitis. Ann Emerg Med 1986;15:557–64.
6. Doria AS, Moineddin R, Kellenberger CJ, et al. US or CT for diagnosis of appendicitis in children and adults? A meta-analysis. Radiology 2006;241:83–94.
7. Solomkin JS, Mazuski JE, Bradley JS, et al. Diagnosis and management of complicated intra-abdominal infection in adults and children: guidelines by the Surgical Infection Society and the Infectious Disease Society of America. Surg Infect (Larchmt) 2010;11:79–109.
8. Lee CC, Golub R, Singer AJ, et al. Routine versus selective abdominal computed tomography scan in the evaluation of right lower quadrant pain: a randomized controlled trial. Acad Emerg Med 2007;14:117–22.
9. McBurney C. Experience with early operative interference in cases of disease of the vermiform appendix. NY Med J 1889;50:676–84.

10. Semm K. Endoscopic appendectomy. Endoscopy 1983;15:59–64.
11. Ingraham AM, Cohen ME, Bilimoria KY, et al. Comparison of outcomes after laparoscopic versus open appendectomy for acute appendicitis at 222 ACS NSQIP hospitals. Surgery 2010;148(4):625–35.
12. Styrud J, Eriksson S, Nilsson I, et al. Appendectomy versus antibiotic treatment in acute appendicitis, a perspective multicenter randomized controlled trial. World J Surg 2006;30:1033–7.
13. Hansson J, Korner U, Khorram-Manesh A, et al. Randomized clinical trial of antibiotic therapy versus appendectomy as primary treatment of acute appendicitis in unselected patients. Br J Surg 2009;96:473–81.
14. Steiner CA, Bass EB, Talamini MA, et al. Surgical rates and operative mortality for open and laparoscopic cholecystectomy in Maryland. N Engl J Med 1994; 330:403–8.
15. Attili AF, Carulli N, Roda E, et al. Epidemiology of gallstone disease in Italy: prevalence data of the Multicenter Italian Study on Cholelithiasis. Am J Epidemiol 1995;141:158–65.
16. Khan KU, Wargo JA. Gallstone disease in the elderly. In: Rosenthal RA, Zenilman ME, Katlie MR, editors. Principles and practice of geriatric surgery. New York: Springer; 2001. p. 690–710.
17. Gurusamy KS, Davidson BR. Surgical treatment of gallstones. Gastroenterol Clin North Am 2010;39:229–44, viii.
18. Portincasa P, Moschetta A, Petruzzelli M, et al. Gallstone disease: symptoms and diagnosis of gallbladder stones. Best Pract Res Clin Gastroenterol 2006; 20:1017–29.
19. Nakeeb A, Ahrendt SA, Pitt HA. Calculus biliary disease. In: Mulholland M, Lillemoe K, Doherty G, et al, editors. Greenfield's surgery: scientific principles and practice. Philadelphia: Lippincott; 2006. p. 978–99.
20. Benarroch-Gampel J, Boyd CA, Sheffield KM, et al. Overuse of CT in patients with complicated gallstone disease. J Am Coll Surg 2011;213:524–30.
21. Tulchinsky M, Colletti PM, Allen TW. Hepatobiliary scintigraphy in acute cholecystitis. Semin Nucl Med 2012;42:84–100.
22. Gurusamy KS, Davidson C, Gluud C, et al. Early versus delayed laparoscopic cholecystectomy for people with acute cholecystitis. Cochrane Database Syst Rev 2013;(6):CD005440.
23. Gurusamy KS, Rossi M, Davidson BR. Percutaneous cholecystotomy for high-risk surgical patients with acute calculous cholecystitis. Cochrane Database Syst Rev 2013;(8):CD007088.
24. Li M, Li N, Ji W, et al. Percutaneous cholecystotomy is a definitive treatment for acute cholecystitis in elderly high-risk patients. Am Surg 2013;79(5):524–7.
25. Jang SE, Park SW, Lee BS, et al. Management for CBD stone-related mild to moderate acute cholangitis: urgent versus elective ERCP. Dig Dis Sci 2013; 58(7):2082–7.
26. Ren Z, Xu Y, Zhu S. Percutaneous transhepatic cholecystotomy for choledocholithiasis with acute cholangitis in high-risk patients. Hepatogastroenterology 2012;59(114):329–31.
27. Navaneethan U, Gutierrez NG, Jegadeesan R, et al. Delay in performing ERCP and adverse events increase the 30-day readmission risk in patients with acute cholangitis. Gastrointest Endosc 2013;78(1):81–90.
28. Natsui M, Saito Y, Abe S, et al. Long-term outcomes of endoscopic papillary balloon dilation and endoscopic sphincterotomy for bile duct stones. Dig Endosc 2013;25(3):313–21.

29. Yasui T, Takahata S, Kono H, et al. Is cholecystectomy necessary after endoscopic treatment of bile duct stones in patients older than 80 years of age? J Gastroenterol 2012;47(1):65–70.

30. Peery AF, Dellon ES, Lund J, et al. Burden of gastrointestinal disease in the United States: 2012 update. Gastroenterology 2012;143(5):1179–87.

31. Fagenholz PJ, Castillo CF, Harris NS, et al. Increasing United States hospital admissions for acute pancreatitis, 1988-2003. Ann Epidemiol 2007;17(7):491–7.

32. Frossard JL, Steer ML, Pastor CM. Acute pancreatitis. Lancet 2008;371(9607): 143–52.

33. Sarr MG, Banks PA, Bollen TL, et al. The new revised classification of acute pancreatitis 2012. Surg Clin North Am 2013;93(3):549–62.

34. Wu BU, Hwang JQ, Gardner TH, et al. Lactated Ringer's solution reduces systemic inflammation compared with saline in patients with acute pancreatitis. Clin Gastroenterol Hepatol 2011;9:710–7.

35. Eckerwall GE, Tingstedt BB, Bergenzaun PE, et al. Immediate oral feeding in patients with mild acute pancreatitis is safe and may accelerate recovery—a randomized clinical study. Clin Nutr 2007;26:758–63.

36. Moraes JM, Felga GE, Chebli LA, et al. A full solid diet as the initial meal in mild acute pancreatitis is safe and results in a shorter length of hospitalization: results from a prospective, randomized, controlled, double-blind clinical trial. J Clin Gastroenterol 2010;44:517–22.

37. Al-Omran M, Albalawi ZH, Tashkandi MF, et al. Enteral versus parenteral nutrition for acute pancreatitis. Cochrane Database Syst Rev 2010;(1):CD002837.

38. Petrov MS, Loveday BP, Pylypchuk RD, et al. Systematic review and meta-analysis of enteral nutrition formulations in acute pancreatitis. Br J Surg 2009; 96:1243–52.

39. Eatock FC, Chong P, Menezes N, et al. A randomized study of early nasogastric versus nasojejunal feeding in severe acute pancreatitis. Am J Gastroenterol 2005;100:432–9.

40. Kumar A, Singh N, Prakash S, et al. Early enteral nutrition in severe acute pancreatitis: a prospective randomized controlled trial comparing nasojejunal and nasogastric routes. J Clin Gastroenterol 2006;40:431–4.

41. Wittau M, Mayer B, Scheele J, et al. Systematic review and meta-analysis of antibiotic prophylaxis in severe acute pancreatitis. Scand J Gastroenterol 2011; 46(3):261–70.

42. Dellinger EP, Tellado JM, Soto NE, et al. Early antibiotic treatment for severe acute necrotizing pancreatitis: randomized, double-blind, placebo-controlled study. Ann Surg 2007;245:674–83.

43. Fleszler F, Friedenberg F, Krevsky B, et al. Abdominal computed tomography prolongs length of stay and is frequently unnecessary in the evaluation of acute pancreatitis. Am J Med Sci 2003;325:251–5.

44. Spanier BW, Nio Y, van der Hulst RW, et al. Practice and yield of early CT scan in acute pancreatitis: a Dutch Observational Multicenter Study. Pancreatology 2010;10:222–8.

45. Mortele KJ, Ip IK, Wu BU, et al. Acute pancreatitis: imaging utilization practices in an urban teaching hospital—analysis of trends with assessment of independent predictors in correlation with patient outcomes. Radiology 2011;258:174–81.

46. Freeman ML, Werner J, van Santvoort HC, et al, International Multidisciplinary Panel of Speakers and Moderators. Interventions for necrotizing pancreatitis: summary of a multidisciplinary consensus conference. Pancreas 2012;41(8): 1176–94.

47. van Santvoort HC, Besselink MG, Bakker OJ, et al, Dutch Pancreatitis Study Group. A step-up approach or open necrosectomy for necrotizing pancreatitis. N Engl J Med 2010;362(16):1491–502.

48. van Santvoort HC, Bakker OJ, Bollen TL, et al, Dutch Pancreatitis Study Group. A conservative and minimally invasive approach to necrotizing pancreatitis improves outcome. Gastroenterology 2011;141(4):1254–63.

49. van Santvoort HC, Besselink MG, Horvath KD, et al, Dutch Acute Pancreatis Study Group. Videoscopic assisted retroperitoneal debridement in infected necrotizing pancreatitis. HPB (Oxford) 2007;9(2):156–9.

50. Bakker OJ, van Santvoort HC, van Brunschot S, et al, Dutch Pancreatitis Study Group. Endoscopic transgastric vs surgical necrosectomy for infected necrotizing pancreatitis: a randomized trial. JAMA 2012;307(10):1053–61.

51. Mantke R, Shulz H, Lippert H. International practices in pancreatic surgery. Part IV, surgery of acute pancreatitis. Berlin (Heidelberg): Springer; 2013.

52. Radenkovic DV, Bajec D, Ivancevic N, et al. Decompressive laparotomy with temporary abdominal closure versus percutaneous puncture with placement of abdominal catheter in patients with abdominal compartment syndrome during acute pancreatitis: background and design of multicenter, randomised, controlled study. BMC Surg 2010;10:22.

53. Boone B, Zureikat A, Hughes SJ, et al. Abdominal compartment syndrome is an early, lethal complication of acute pancreatitis. Am Surg 2013;79(6):601–7.

54. Kalva SP, Yeddula K, Wicky S, et al. Angiographic intervention in patients with a suspected visceral artery pseudoaneurysm complicating pancreatitis and pancreatic surgery. Arch Surg 2011;146(6):647–52.

55. Samuelson AL, Shah RJ. Endoscopic management of pancreatic pseudocysts. Gastroenterol Clin North Am 2012;41(1):47–62.

56. Besselink MG. Splanchnic vein thrombosis complicating severe acute pancreatitis. HPB (Oxford) 2011;13(12):831–2.

57. Nguyen GC, Sam J, Anand N. Epidemiological trends and geographic variation in hospital admissions for diverticulitis in the United States. World J Gastroenterol 2011;17(12):1600–5.

58. Shahedi K, Fuller G, Bolus R, et al. Long-term risk of acute diverticulitis among patients with incidental diverticulosis found during colonoscopy. Clin Gastroenterol Hepatol 2013. [Epub ahead of print].

59. Rafferty J, Shellito P, Hyman NH, et al, Standards Committee of American Society of Colon and Rectal Surgeons. Practice parameters for sigmoid diverticulitis. Dis Colon Rectum 2006;49(7):939–44.

60. Humes DJ, West J. Role of acute diverticulitis in the development of complicated colonic diverticular disease and 1-year mortality after diagnosis in the UK: population-based cohort study. Gut 2012;61(1):95–100.

61. Touzios JG, Dozois EJ. Diverticulosis and acute diverticulitis. Gastroenterol Clin North Am 2009;38(3):513–25.

62. Commane DM, Arasaradnam RP, Mills S, et al. Diet, ageing and genetic factors in the pathogenesis of diverticular disease. World J Gastroenterol 2009;15(20): 2479–88.

63. Chabok A, Påhlman L, Hjern F, et al, AVOD Study Group. Randomized clinical trial of antibiotics in acute uncomplicated diverticulitis. Br J Surg 2012;99(4): 532–9.

64. Solomkin JS. Evaluating evidence and grading recommendations: the SIS/IDSA guidelines for the treatment of complicated intra-abdominal infections. Surg Infect (Larchmt) 2010;11(3):269–74.

65. Brandt D, Gervaz P, Durmishi Y, et al. Percutaneous CT scan-guided drainage vs. antibiotherapy alone for Hinchey II diverticulitis: a case-control study. Dis Colon Rectum 2006;49(10):1533.
66. Siewert B, Tye G, Kruskal J, et al. Impact of CT-guided drainage in the treatment of diverticular abscesses: size matters. AJR Am J Roentgenol 2006; 186(3):680.
67. Kam MH, Tang CL, Chan E, et al. Systematic review of intraoperative colonic irrigation vs. manual decompression in obstructed left-sided colorectal emergencies. Int J Colorectal Dis 2009;24(9):1031–7.
68. Jiménez Fuertes M, Costa Navarro D. Resection and primary anastomosis without diverting ileostomy for left colon emergencies: is it a safe procedure? World J Surg 2012;36(5):1148–53.
69. Forshaw MJ, Sankararajah D, Stewart M, et al. Self-expanding metallic stents in the treatment of benign colorectal disease: indications and outcomes. Colorectal Dis 2006;8(2):102–11.
70. Costi R, Cauchy F, Le Bian A, et al. Challenging a classic myth: pneumoperitoneum associated with acute diverticulitis is not an indication for open or laparoscopic emergency surgery in hemodynamically stable patients. A 10-year experience with a nonoperative treatment. Surg Endosc 2012;26(7):2061–71.
71. Oberkofler CE, Rickenbacher A, Raptis DA, et al. A multicenter randomized clinical trial of primary anastomosis or Hartmann's procedure for perforated left colonic diverticulitis with purulent or fecal peritonitis. Ann Surg 2012;256(5): 819–26.
72. Afshar S, Kurer MA. Laparoscopic peritoneal lavage for perforated sigmoid diverticulitis. Colorectal Dis 2012;14(2):135–42.
73. Lau KC, Spilsbury K, Farooque Y, et al. Is colonoscopy still mandatory after a CT diagnosis of left-sided diverticulitis: can colorectal cancer be confidently excluded? Dis Colon Rectum 2011;54(10):1265–70.
74. Ünlü C, Daniels L, Vrouenraets BC, et al. A systematic review of high-fibre dietary therapy in diverticular disease. Int J Colorectal Dis 2012;27(4):419–27.
75. Unlü C, Daniels L, Vrouenraets BC, et al. Systematic review of medical therapy to prevent recurrent diverticulitis. Int J Colorectal Dis 2012;27(9):1131–6.
76. Tursi A, Brandimarte G, Daffinà R. Long-term treatment with mesalazine and rifaximin versus rifaximin alone for patients with recurrent attacks of acute diverticulitis of colon. Dig Liver Dis 2002;34(7):510–5.
77. Kaiser AM, Jiang JK, Lake JP, et al. The management of complicated diverticulitis and the role of computed tomography. Am J Gastroenterol 2005;100(4): 910–7.
78. Gaertner WB, Willis DJ, Madoff RD, et al. Percutaneous drainage of colonic diverticular abscess: is colon resection necessary? Dis Colon Rectum 2013; 56(5):622–6.
79. Klarenbeek BR, Veenhof AA, Bergamaschi R, et al. Laparoscopic sigmoid resection for diverticulitis decreases major morbidity rates: a randomized control trial: short-term results of the Sigma Trial. Ann Surg 2009;249(1):39–44.
80. Ricciardi R, Rothenberger DA, Madoff RD, et al. Increasing prevalence and severity of *Clostridium difficile* colitis in hospitalized patients in the United States. Arch Surg 2007;142(7):624–31 [discussion: 631].
81. Lucado J, Gould C, Elishauser A. *Clostridium difficile* infections (CDI) in hospital stays, 2009. HCUP statistical brief no. 124. 2011.
82. U.S. Department of Health and Human Services AfHRaQ. HCUP projections; *Clostridium difficile* infection 2011 to 2012. 2012.

83. Sailhamer EA, Carson K, Chang Y, et al. Fulminant *Clostridium difficile* colitis: patterns of care and predictors of mortality. Arch Surg 2009;144(5):433–9 [discussion: 439–40].

84. Byrn JC, Maun DC, Gingold DS, et al. Predictors of mortality after colectomy for fulminant *Clostridium difficile* colitis. Arch Surg 2008;143(2):150–4 [discussion: 155].

85. Bartlett JG. Narrative review: the new epidemic of *Clostridium difficile*-associated enteric disease. Ann Intern Med 2006;145(10):758–64.

86. Loo VG, Bourgault AM, Poirier L, et al. Host and pathogen factors for *Clostridium difficile* infection and colonization. N Engl J Med 2011;365(18):1693–703.

87. Siegel JD, Rhinehart E, Jackson M, et al. Healthcare Infection Control Practices Advisory Committee 2007 guideline for isolation precautions: preventing transmission of infectious agents in healthcare settings. 2007. Available at: http://www.cdc.gov/ncidod/dhqp/gl_isolation.html. Accessed May 10, 2013.

88. Cohen SH, Gerding DN, Johnson S, et al, Society for Healthcare Epidemiology of America, Infectious Diseases Society of America. Clinical practice guidelines for *Clostridium difficile* infection in adults: 2010 update by the Society for Healthcare Epidemiology of America (SHEA) and the Infectious Diseases Society of America (IDSA). Infect Control Hosp Epidemiol 2010;31(5):431.

89. Louie TJ, Miller MA, Mullane KM, et al, OPT-80-003 Clinical Study Group. Fidaxomicin versus vancomycin for *Clostridium difficile* infection. N Engl J Med 2011;364(5):422–31.

90. McFarland LV. Alternative treatments for *Clostridium difficile* disease: what really works? J Med Microbiol 2005;54(Pt 2):101.

91. Cornely OA, Miller MA, Louie TJ, et al. Treatment of first recurrence of *Clostridium difficile* infection: fidaxomicin versus vancomycin. Clin Infect Dis 2012;55(Suppl 2):S154–61.

92. McFarland LV, Elmer GW, Surawicz CM. Breaking the cycle: treatment strategies for 163 cases of recurrent *Clostridium difficile* disease. Am J Gastroenterol 2002;97(7):1769.

93. van Nood E, Vrieze A, Nieuwdorp M, et al. Duodenal infusion of donor feces for recurrent *Clostridium difficile*. N Engl J Med 2013;368(5):407–15.

94. Koss K, Clark MA, Sanders DS, et al. The outcome of surgery in fulminant *Clostridium difficile* colitis. Colorectal Dis 2006;8(2):149.

95. Neal MD, Alverdy JC, Hall DE, et al. Diverting loop ileostomy and colonic lavage: an alternative to total abdominal colectomy for the treatment of severe, complicated *Clostridium difficile* associated disease. Ann Surg 2011;254(3):423–7 [discussion: 427–9].

96. Lowy I, Molrine DC, Leav BA, et al. Treatment with monoclonal antibodies against *Clostridium difficile* toxins. N Engl J Med 2010;362(3):197.

Gastroduodenal Perforation

Raminder Nirula, MD, MPH

KEYWORDS

• Gastroduodenal • Perforation • Ulcer-reducing surgery

KEY POINTS

- The most common cause of gastroduodenal perforation is peptic ulcer disease.
- Nonoperative management can be considered in patients with minimal symptoms who are younger than 70 years.
- Abdominal washout, ulcer biopsy, and omental patch are appropriate in most circumstances.
- Acid-reducing surgery is indicated in patients who have a history of failed medical therapy.

The cause and management of gastroduodenal perforation has changed as a result of increasing use of nonsteroidal antiinflammatories and improved pharmacologic treatment of acid hypersecretion, as well as the recognition and treatment of *Helicobacter pylori* (**Fig. 1**). As a result of the reduction in ulcer recurrence with medical therapy, the surgical approach to patients with gastroduodenal perforation has also changed over the last 3 decades, with ulcer-reducing surgery being performed infrequently.[1,2]

CAUSE

- The most common cause of gastroduodenal perforation is ulcer disease
  - Ulcer disease may be secondary to acid hypersecretion, *H pylori* infection, or from medications (steroids, nonsteroidal antiinflammatories)
- Other causes include trauma, neoplasm, foreign body ingestion, or iatrogenic (endoscopic procedures).
  - Blunt trauma resulting in gastroduodenal perforation is rare, comprising only 5% of blunt hollow viscous injuries.
  - Malignant perforations may be secondary to necrotic tumor in the stomach or duodenum that perforates or from an obstructing tumor, leading to proximal dilation and perforation.
  - Foreign bodies may cause perforation from direct injury to the stomach or duodenum or as a result of luminal obstruction.[1]

Department of Surgery, University of Utah, 50 North Medical Drive, Salt Lake City, UT 84132, USA
E-mail address: r.nirula@hsc.utah.edu

Surg Clin N Am 94 (2014) 31–34
http://dx.doi.org/10.1016/j.suc.2013.10.002   surgical.theclinics.com
0039-6109/14/$ – see front matter © 2014 Elsevier Inc. All rights reserved.

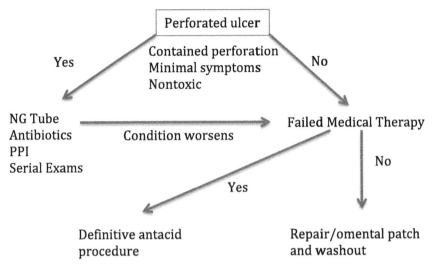

Fig. 1. Treatment of perforated gastroduodenal ulcer. Exams, examinations; NG, nasogastric; PPI, proton pump inhibitor.

PRESENTATION

- Sudden onset of severe epigastric and right upper quadrant abdominal pain in patients with a history of gastroesophageal reflux is common among those with peptic ulcer disease perforations.
- Peritonitis may be minimal in the case of contained leaks.
- Mental status changes and septic shock (fever, hypotension, tachycardia) may be observed in diffuse leakage of the perforation.

DIAGNOSIS

- Leukocytosis, metabolic acidosis, and hyperamylasemia may be present but are not sensitive.
- Upright chest radiograph may show free air.
- Computed tomography (CT) with enteral contrast shows free air, free fluid, mesenteric fat stranding, and bowel wall thickening and may localize the site of perforation. Early CT scans after traumatic injury may be falsely negative in up to 12% of cases.[3]

MANAGEMENT
Nonoperative Management

Approximately half of the perforations spontaneously seal, which raises the question as to whether these patients can be managed nonoperatively. The difficulty is identifying those patients who have sealed without compromising the outcomes for those who have not sealed while one observes them for signs of clinical deterioration.[4] Factors mandating surgical management include shock and generalized peritonitis. Risk factors that have been associated with failure of nonoperative management include age greater than 70 years, symptoms of greater than 24 hours, and lack of improvement after 12 hours of conservative therapy. Conservative therapy includes showing that there is no free extravasation of contrast and that the leak is confined either by CT or gastroduodenography. Once this information is verified, a nasogastric tube for decompression is required. The patient should receive antimicrobial therapy directed at aerobic gram-positive cocci such as ampicillin/sulbactam, as well as a proton pump inhibitor.[5] Should the patient fail to improve or worsen (fever, shock, worsening peritonitis), prompt surgical intervention is required.

Operative Management

Patients who have free perforation, shock, generalized peritonitis, or progressive symptoms should undergo surgery. The decision to perform an acid-reducing operation is made based on the patient's history. Those patients who have perforated despite antacid therapy and H pylori eradication or who require ulcerogenic medications such as steroids should undergo an acid-reducing operation. For those who have not received adequate medical therapy, ulcer biopsy for gastric ulcers, omental patch, and abdominal washout followed by medical therapy provide acceptably low ulcer recurrence rates, of less then 10%.[6–8]

In patients who have failed medical therapy and are hemodynamically stable, there are several antacid operations, each with its merits: truncal vagotomy with pyloroplasty, truncal vagotomy with antrectomy, and either a Bilroth I or Bilroth II reconstruction, or highly selective vagotomy. These operations should generally be reserved for ulcers that are related to acid hypersecretion, which include prepyloric ulcers or gastric ulcers within the body that occur in conjunction with duodenal ulcers. The choice of which operation to perform needs to take into account the location of the perforation and the ability to achieve closure along with the risk for ulcer recurrence balanced by the risk of complications related to the operation. Vagotomy and antrectomy carries the lowest risk for ulcer recurrence, at approximately 2%, whereas vagotomy and pyloroplasty carries a recurrence rate of 5%, and 10% to 20% for highly selective vagotomy.[9,10]

Closure of gastric perforations can typically be easily performed, because of the mobility and redundancy of the stomach, which can then be reinforced with an omental patch. Duodenal perforations frequently cannot be primarily closed unless they are small without causing duodenal narrowing. Therefore, an omental or jejunal serosal patch may be necessary. If the integrity of the repair is in question, the right upper quadrant should be drained in anticipation of a duodenal fistula and a gastrostomy tube for drainage, and a jejunal feeding tube should be placed. In patients who are hemodynamically normal, this procedure may be performed laparoscopically. If the perforation is proximal and an antacid operation is being performed, then, the ulcer may be resected if the remaining duodenal stump is not indurated, and the resection can be performed without injury to the ampulla.

REFERENCES

1. Lui FY, Davis KA. Gastroduodenal perforation: maximal or minimal intervention? Scand J Surg 2010;99(2):73–7.
2. Meissner K. H2-receptor antagonists and the incidence of gastroduodenal ulcer perforation and hemorrhage. An epidemiological study. Chirurg 1990;61(6):449–52 [discussion: 453]. [in German].
3. Fakhry SM, Watts DD, Luchette FA. Current diagnostic approaches lack sensitivity in the diagnosis of perforated blunt small bowel injury: analysis from 275,557 trauma admissions from the EAST multi-institutional HVI trial. J Trauma 2003;54(2):295–306.
4. Crofts TJ, Park KG, Steele RJ, et al. A randomized trial of nonoperative treatment for perforated peptic ulcer. N Engl J Med 1989;320(15):970–3.

5. Solomkin JS, Mazuski JE, Bradley JS, et al. Diagnosis and management of complicated intra-abdominal infection in adults and children: guidelines by the Surgical Infection Society and the Infectious Diseases Society of America. Clin Infect Dis 2010;50(2):133–64.

6. Wong BC, Lam SK, Lai KC, et al. Triple therapy for *Helicobacter pylori* eradication is more effective than long-term maintenance antisecretory treatment in the prevention of recurrence of duodenal ulcer: a prospective long-term follow-up study. Aliment Pharmacol Ther 1999;13(3):303–9.

7. Axon AT, O'Morain CA, Bardhan KD, et al. Randomised double blind controlled study of recurrence of gastric ulcer after treatment for eradication of *Helicobacter pylori* infection. BMJ 1997;314(7080):565–8.

8. Graham DY, Lew GM, Klein PD, et al. Effect of treatment of *Helicobacter pylori* infection on the long-term recurrence of gastric or duodenal ulcer. A randomized, controlled study. Ann Intern Med 1992;116(9):705–8.

9. Busman DC, Volovics A, Munting JD. Recurrence rate after highly selective vagotomy. World J Surg 1988;12(2):217–23.

10. Sawyer JL, Scott HW Jr. Selective gastric vagotomy with antrectomy or pyloroplasty. Ann Surg 1971;174(4):541–7.

Esophageal Perforation

Raminder Nirula, MD, MPH

KEYWORDS

- Esophageal perforation • Sepsis • Iatrogenic perforation • Management

KEY POINTS

- Esophageal perforation most frequently occurs secondary to endoscopically induced injury.
- Patients may progress quickly to septic shock, which mandates immediate surgical intervention.
- Thoracic-contained perforations may be managed nonoperatively if patients are not septic and imaging shows a contained perforation.
- Esophageal stenting has been effective in patients with malignancy-associated perforation.
- Primary repair and drainage should be used in patients without malignancy.

Esophageal perforation is relatively uncommon but carries a high morbidity and mortality (10%–40%), particularly if the injury is not detected early before the onset of systemic signs of sepsis.[1,2] The fact that it is an uncommon problem and it produces symptoms that can mimic other serious thoracic conditions, such as myocardial infarction, contributes to the delay in diagnosis. Furthermore, patients at risk for iatrogenic perforations (esophageal malignancy) frequently have comorbidities that increase their perioperative morbidity and mortality.[3] The optimal treatment of esophageal perforation varies with respect to the time of presentation, the extent of the perforation, and the underlying esophageal pathologic condition.

CAUSE

- The most common cause is iatrogenic at sites of luminal narrowing during endoscopy (cricopharyngeus, aortic knob, gastroesophageal junction and pathologic sites such as tumors or strictures).[4] Therefore, underlying conditions are frequently present, which lead to the endoscopically induced injury (**Box 1**).
- The classic description is a perforation that occurs spontaneously after vomiting, as described by Boerhaave, in which the tear occurs in the distal esophagus.

Department of Surgery, University of Utah, 50 North Medical Drive, Salt Lake City, UT 84132, USA
E-mail address: r.nirula@hsc.utah.edu

Surg Clin N Am 94 (2014) 35–41
http://dx.doi.org/10.1016/j.suc.2013.10.003
0039-6109/14/$ – see front matter © 2014 Elsevier Inc. All rights reserved.

surgical.theclinics.com

Box 1
Common conditions associated with esophageal perforation

Malignancy

Gastroesophageal reflux disease

Achalasia

Stricture (eg, caustic, benign, anastamotic)

Scleroderma

Hiatal hernia

- Blunt trauma to the epigastrium can cause distal esophageal perforation, although this is rare. Penetrating trauma can result in injury anywhere in the esophagus but is frequently associated with trauma to the surrounding structures.
- Ingestion of caustic substances can lead to full-thickness perforation.

PRESENTATION

- Pain is the most frequent complaint.
  - ○ Cervical esophageal perforation results in dysphagia, or pain with neck flexion may be noted.
  - ○ Thoracic esophageal perforation presents with pain in the back, chest, or epigastrium. Most of these injuries occur on the distal left side of the esophagus because there is little protection from surrounding structures.
  - ○ Distal injuries that leak into the abdomen will lead to abdominal pain and peritonitis. Epigastric pain may radiate to the shoulders because of diaphragmatic irritation.
- Other symptoms that are less frequently observed include dysphagia, hematemesis, and nausea/vomiting (**Table 1**).

Table 1
Signs and symptoms of esophageal perforation

Sign or Symptom	Frequency (%)
Pain	70
Dyspnea	26
Fever	44
Emphysema	25
Pneumomediastinum	19
Nausea or vomiting	19
Pneumothorax	14
Pleural effusion	14
Hematemesis	8
Dysphagia	12
Empyema	8

Data from Hasimoto CN, Cataneo C, Eldib R, et al. Efficacy of surgical versus conservative treatment in esophageal perforation: a systematic review of case series studies. Acta Cir Bras 2013;28(4):266–71.

- Crepitus on the chest or neck may be palpable because of subcutaneous emphysema.
- Systemic signs of infection/inflammation include fever, tachycardia, and eventual hypotension.

DIAGNOSIS

- Chest radiography findings include mediastinal air, pleural effusion, pneumothorax, and subdiaphragmatic air.
- Chest tube output may contain particulate matter or acidic fluid.
- Meglumine diatrizoate (Gastrografin) is generally accepted as the first agent that should be used to assess for perforation instead of barium to avoid the inflammatory reaction of barium. A false-negative rate of as much as 10% may be seen with Gastrografin; therefore, if suspicion remains high in the setting of a nondiagnostic study, thin barium may then be used.
- Because most perforations are associated with endoscopy, repeat endoscopy as a diagnostic procedure should be avoided; however, it has some diagnostic and therapeutic utility if the perforation is suspected to be secondary to malignancy. Endoscopy should not be used for diagnostic purposes in unstable patients because these patients likely need surgical debridement, and their perforation site should be identifiable via radiographic means.
- Computed tomography scan may reveal contrast extravasation as well as loculated fluid collections that can facilitate the management decisions in terms of a percutaneous approach for drainage versus wide operative debridement.

MANAGEMENT

Patients with esophageal perforation can quickly progress to septic shock and, therefore, should be closely monitored. The principles of the management of esophageal perforation should primarily focus on source control and secondarily consider the underlying disease process (**Fig. 1**). Abdominal esophageal perforations should be managed surgically because leakage will be free into the peritoneal cavity making conservative therapy ineffective.

At a minimum, broad-spectrum antibiotic therapy should be administered early, and a chest tube should be inserted to drain effusions and/or pneumothoraces while the therapeutic approach is being determined. Plans for parenteral nutrition should be made until enteral nutrition can be delivered safely.

Nonoperative Management

Approximately one-quarter of patients can be managed nonoperatively and consists of patients who have no signs of systemic infection/sepsis and have features that are associated with a high rate of success for nonoperative management (**Box 2**). Patients should be given nothing by mouth for a minimum of 7 days and then have a Gastrografin swallow to determine if the leak has sealed. If the leak remains but patients show no signs of clinical deterioration, this approach can be continued with repeat contrast studies weekly until there is resolution of the leak, at which point enteral nutrition can be reinitiated. If the clinical condition deteriorates, operative intervention is necessary.

Several series have examined the efficacy of esophageal stenting for perforation primarily in the setting of malignant perforation or in postoperative patients with an anastomotic leak. In a series of 19 patients with spontaneous esophageal perforation, 89% had occlusion of their leaks with stenting and adequate drainage; the 2 patients who failed both had perforations extending across the gastroesophageal junction that

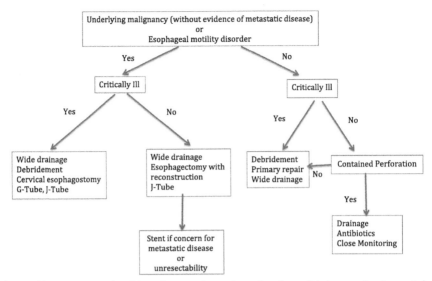

Fig. 1. Management algorithm for esophageal perforation. G-tube, gastrostomy tube; J-tube, Jejunostomy tube.

required surgical intervention. Most patients resumed enteral nutrition within 3 days of the stent placement. Approximately one-fifth of the patients had stent migration requiring repeat endoscopic manipulation.[5] Similar success rates have been observed in series that use stenting for esophageal anastomotic leaks.[6–8]

Identifying patients likely to fail stent therapy would hasten a surgical approach if warranted, thus avoiding delays in obtaining source control. A study of 187 patients having stents placed for esophageal leaks demonstrated that those who failed to achieve source control from stenting were more likely to have a cervical leak, a leak spanning the gastroesophageal junction, or an injury longer then 6 cm.[9] Such patients should, therefore, be considered for a surgical approach rather then stenting.

Operative Management

The surgical options include the following:
- Drainage of the contaminated space
- Debridement with primary repair of the perforation

Box 2
Factors associated with success of nonoperative management

Recent perforation

Well-circumscribed perforation

Not perforated within the abdominal cavity

Contained cavity that drains back into esophagus

No free extravasation of contrast into body cavities

No malignancy, obstruction, or stricture in region of perforation

No evidence of sepsis

Minimal symptoms

- Esophageal diversion and delayed repair
- Esophagectomy

Drainage of the Contaminated Space

Drainage of the pleural space was traditionally thought to be suitable as the sole treatment of esophageal perforations in the minority of patients; however, there are at least 3 series that have reported low mortality rates for this treatment option. Mengoli and colleagues[10] reported a 6% mortality in their series of 21 patients managed without thoracotomy. Martinez and colleagues[11] reported a 100% survival in their pediatric series of iatrogenic perforations with an algorithm that involved pleural drainage but not immediate surgical debridement. A similar series of 34 patents published by Vogel and colleagues[12] had 2 deaths out of 6 undergoing operative procedures and no deaths in the conservatively treated group with radiographically demonstrated healing in 96%.

These series suggest that in appropriately selected patients, pleural drainage, antibiotics, and parenteral nutrition in stable patients may achieve acceptable mortality rates as good as or superior to operative intervention.

Primary Repair

For patients with iatrogenic perforation or Boerhaave, primary repair is appropriate. Traditionally, primary repair was only appropriate for patients who presented within 24 hours of their perforation because of the worse outcomes being reported for those presenting beyond 24 hours.[13] With improved surgical critical care, several series have reported equivalent mortality for patients undergoing primary repair beyond 24 hours of the perforation, justifying this approach.[14–17] A 27-year, single-center, retrospective review of 119 patients, with the majority having thoracic perforations, showed that most of the benign perforations were repaired primarily. A third of the malignant thoracic perforations were managed with a chest tube alone or in conjunction with an expandable stent. Because the sample sizes were small, mortality rates for primary repair, resection and reconstruction, diversion, drainage alone, or drainage with stenting were not statistically different. Their analysis included a multivariate regression model to identify independent predictors of mortality, which included the preoperative need for mechanical ventilation, malignant perforation, a Charlson comorbidity index of 7.1 or greater, preexisting pulmonary disease, and presentation with sepsis.[3]

Primary repair should include esophagomyotomy proximal and distal to the tear, debridement of necrotic tissue, reapproximation of the esophageal mucosa, buttressing of the esophageal musculature over the perforation site, and tissue flaps of pleura or intercostal muscle if in the chest or strap muscles if in the neck. A feeding jejunostomy and draining gastrostomy may be placed during the primary repair, which will be extremely useful should the primary repair fail.

Esophageal Diversion and Delayed Repair

In patients with significantly devitalized tissue that precludes primary repair or when primary repair has failed and source control is necessary because of ongoing mediastinal sepsis, esophageal diversion and delayed repair is recommended. Typically in this scenario, esophagectomy is unsafe because patients are in septic shock and a prolonged procedure will lead to death in the operating room. Therefore, source control via debridement, drainage, and proximal diversion via a cervical esophagostomy is warranted. Gastrostomy and feeding jejunostomy are important to allow for distal drainage and feeding. Several months after resolution of the mediastinal sepsis, reconstruction can be performed with either gastric or colonic interposition.

Esophagectomy

Resection should be considered if the perforation is in conjunction with esophageal malignancy, a distal esophageal stricture, esophageal necrosis as with caustic inges-tion, or esophageal motility disorders that would lead to poor healing of a primary repair, such as achalasia. In cases when there is significant mediastinal/pleural contamination, a transthoracic approach should be undertaken to ensure adequate debridement. But in early iatrogenic cases, the degree of contamination and necrosis is less; therefore, a transhiatal esophagectomy may be performed. Restoration of intestinal continuity should only be undertaken at the first operation if patients are not critically ill.

REFERENCES

1. Reeder LB, DeFilippi VJ, Ferguson MK. Current results of therapy for esophageal perforation. Am J Surg 1995;169(6):615–7.
2. Muir AD, White J, McGuigan JA, et al. Treatment and outcomes of oesophageal perforation in a tertiary referral centre. Eur J Cardiothorac Surg 2003;23(5): 799–804 [discussion: 804].
3. Bhatia P, Fortin D, Inculet RI, et al. Current concepts in the management of esophageal perforations: a twenty-seven year Canadian experience. Ann Thorac Surg 2011;92(1):209–15.
4. Hasimoto CN, Cataneo C, Eldib R, et al. Efficacy of surgical versus conservative treatment in esophageal perforation: a systematic review of case series studies. Acta Cir Bras 2013;28(4):266–71.
5. Freeman RK, Van Woerkom JM, Vyverberg A, et al. Esophageal stent placement for the treatment of spontaneous esophageal perforations. Ann Thorac Surg 2009;88(1):194–8.
6. Dai Y, Chopra SS, Kneif S, et al. Management of esophageal anastomotic leaks, perforations, and fistulae with self-expanding plastic stents. J Thorac Cardiovasc Surg 2011;141(5):1213–7.
7. Salminen P, Gullichsen R, Laine S. Use of self-expandable metal stents for the treatment of esophageal perforations and anastomotic leaks. Surg Endosc 2009;23(7):1526–30.
8. Tuebergen D, Rijcken E, Mennigen R, et al. Treatment of thoracic esopha-geal anastomotic leaks and esophageal perforations with endoluminal stents: efficacy and current limitations. J Gastrointest Surg 2008;12(7): 1168–76.
9. Freeman RK, Ascioti AJ, Giannini T, et al. Analysis of unsuccessful esophageal stent placements for esophageal perforation, fistula, or anastomotic leak. Ann Thorac Surg 2012;94(3):959–64 [discussion 964–5].
10. Mengoli LR, Klassen KP. Conservative management of esophageal perforation. Arch Surg 1965;91:238.
11. Martinez L, Rivas S, Hernández F, et al. Aggressive conservative treat-ment of esophageal perforations in children. J Pediatr Surg 2003;38(5): 685–9.
12. Vogel SB, Rout WR, Martin TD, et al. Esophageal perforation in adults: aggres-sive, conservative treatment lowers morbidity and mortality. Ann Surg 2005; 241(6):1016–21 [discussion: 1021–3].
13. Salo JA, Isolauri JO, Heikkila LJ, et al. Management of delayed esophageal perforation with mediastinal sepsis. Esophagectomy or primary repair? J Thorac Cardiovasc Surg 1993;106(6):1088–91.

14. Jougon J, Mc Bride T, Delcambre F, et al. Primary esophageal repair for Boerhaave's syndrome whatever the free interval between perforation and treatment. Eur J Cardiothorac Surg 2004;25(4):475–9.
15. Sung SW, Park JJ, Kim YT, et al. Surgery in thoracic esophageal perforation: primary repair is feasible. Dis Esophagus 2002;15(3):204–9.
16. Bardaxoglou E, Manganas D, Meunier B, et al. New approach to surgical management of early esophageal thoracic perforation: primary suture repair reinforced with absorbable mesh and fibrin glue. World J Surg 1997;21(6):618–21.
17. Wang N, Razzouk AJ, Safavi A, et al. Delayed primary repair of intrathoracic esophageal perforation: is it safe? J Thorac Cardiovasc Surg 1996;111(1):114–21 [discussion: 121–2].

Upper Gastrointestinal Bleeding

Marcie Feinman, MD, Elliott R. Haut, MD*

KEYWORDS

- Upper gastrointestinal bleeding • Ulcer disease • Gastroesophageal varices
- Endoscopy

KEY POINTS

- Upper gastrointestinal (GI) bleeding remains a commonly encountered diagnosis for acute care surgeons.
- Initial stabilization and resuscitation of patients is imperative.
- Stable patients can have initiation of medical therapy and localization of the bleeding, whereas persistently unstable patients require emergent endoscopic or operative intervention.
- Minimally invasive techniques have surpassed surgery as the treatment of choice for most upper GI bleeding.

INTRODUCTION

Acute gastrointestinal (GI) bleeding can run the gamut from mild to immediately life-threatening. It has an incidence of 100 cases per 100,000 population per year, and remains a common cause of hospitalization and consultation among acute care surgeons.

GI bleeding is defined as upper or lower, based on the relationship to the ligament of Treitz. The source in upper GI bleeding is proximal to the ligament of Treitz and is associated with a mortality of 6% to 10%. Mortality is often based on the underlying cause as well as patient comorbidities. Sung and colleagues[1] determined that most patients with bleeding from peptic ulcer disease (80%) died of non–bleeding-related causes.

BLOOD SUPPLY OF THE FOREGUT

Upper GI bleeding can involve the esophagus, stomach, and/or duodenum. These structures have a rich vascular supply that can cause life-threatening exsanguination if large vessels are disrupted.

Division of Acute Care Surgery, Department of Surgery, Anesthesiology/Critical Care Medicine (ACCM), Emergency Medicine, The Johns Hopkins University School of Medicine, Sheikh Zayed Tower, 1800 Orleans Street, Suite 6017, Baltimore, MD 21287, USA
* Corresponding author.
E-mail address: ehaut1@jhmi.edu

Surg Clin N Am 94 (2014) 43–53
http://dx.doi.org/10.1016/j.suc.2013.10.004
0039-6109/14/$ – see front matter © 2014 Elsevier Inc. All rights reserved.
surgical.theclinics.com

Esophagus

The upper esophageal sphincter and cervical esophagus get their blood supply from the inferior thyroid artery. The thoracic esophagus is supplied by paired aortic esophageal arteries or branches of the bronchial arteries while the distal esophagus and lower esophageal sphincter are perfused by the left gastric artery and left phrenic artery (**Fig. 1**).

Stomach

The stomach has a redundant blood supply from multiple vessels. The lesser curvature contains the right and left gastric arteries while the greater curve is supplied by

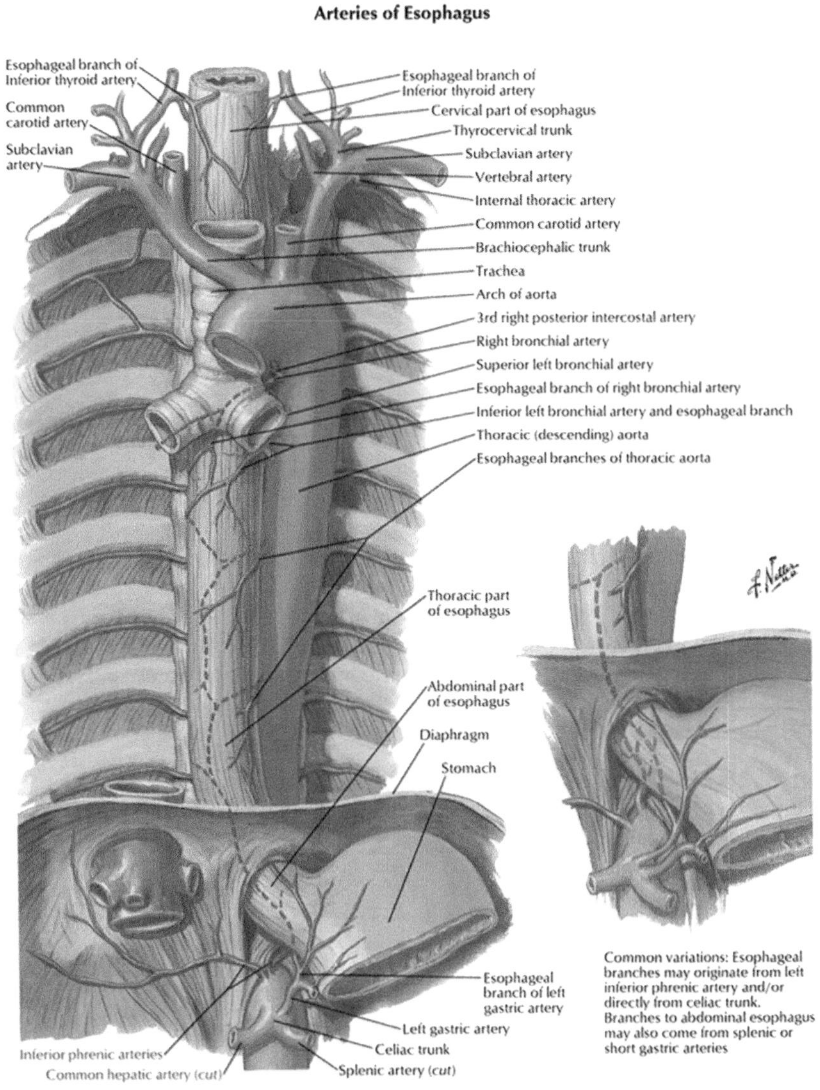

Arteries of Esophagus

Fig. 1. Arteries of the esophagus. (Netter illustration from www.netterimages.com. © Elsevier Inc. All rights reserved.)

the right and left gastroepiploic arteries. The short gastric arteries arise from the splenic artery and contribute to perfusion of the gastric fundus.

Duodenum

The duodenum receives its blood supply from branches of 2 major arteries: the celiac trunk and the superior mesenteric artery (SMA). The first and second portions of the duodenum are perfused mainly via the gastroduodenal artery (GDA) and its branch, the superior pancreaticoduodenal artery. The GDA originates from the hepatic artery off the celiac trunk. The third and fourth portions of the duodenum receive blood supply from the inferior pancreaticoduodenal artery, which is a branch of the SMA (**Fig. 2**).

ETIOLOGY AND PATHOPHYSIOLOGY

Upper GI bleeding has many causes, each with unique pathophysiology and management challenges; the most common are described here.

Peptic Ulcer Disease

Gastric and duodenal ulcers are the most common cause of upper GI bleeding. Ninety percent of duodenal ulcers and 70% of gastric ulcers are associated with *Helicobacter pylori*. Identified in 1982, this gram-negative bacterium disrupts the mucosal barrier and causes inflammation of the mucosa of the stomach and duodenum. Another common

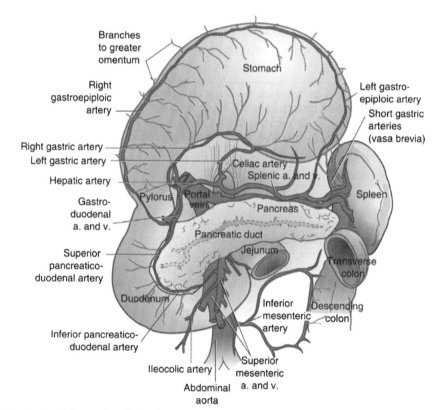

Fig. 2. Arterial supply of the foregut. (*From* Zuidema G. Shackelford's Surgery of the Alimentary Tract, 4th edition. Philadelphia: WB Saunders; 1995; with permission.)

cause of peptic ulcer disease is nonsteroidal anti-inflammatory drugs (NSAIDs), which inhibit cyclooxygenase, leading to impaired mucosal defenses via decreased mucosal prostaglandin synthesis. Use of NSAIDs has a more pronounced effect on the stomach than on the duodenum, with a 40-fold increase in gastric ulcers and an 8-fold increase in duodenal ulcers. Approximately 20% of long-term NSAID users will have mucosal ulceration.[2] Regardless of etiology, as the ulcer progresses beyond the mucosa to the submucosa the inflammation causes weakening and necrosis of arterial walls, leading to pseudoaneurysm formation followed by rupture and hemorrhage. The severity of the bleed is directly related to the size of the involved vessels.

Mallory-Weiss Tear

Responsible for up to 15% of upper GI bleeds, Mallory-Weiss tears consist of longitudinal lacerations in the cardia of the stomach or gastroesophageal (GE) junction.[3] These tears were first reported in 1929 by Mallory and Weiss, and were initially described in association with vomiting following an alcoholic binge.[4] The definition has since been expanded to include any event that causes a sudden increase in intragastric pressure.

Stress Gastritis

The mucosa of the stomach is protected from the acidic environment by mucus, bicarbonate, prostaglandins, and blood flow. If the balance of gastric acid secretion and mucosal defenses is disrupted, acid interacts with the epithelium to cause damage. In stress gastritis, there is no evidence of acid hypersecretion; therefore, the breakdown of mucosal defenses leads to injury of the mucosa and subsequent bleeding.[5] Two classically described patient populations in which this is seen are those with elevated intracranial pressure (Cushing ulcer) and major burns (Curling ulcer).

Dieulafoy Lesion

Dieulafoy lesions are large, tortuous, histologically normal vessels located in the submucosa. These vessels often protrude through mucosal defects, rendering them at risk for rupture because of necrosis of the arterial wall from exposure to gastric acid.[6] These lesions are found most often within 6 cm of the GE junction on the lesser curve of the stomach.

Gastroesophageal Varices

A result of portal hypertension, GE varices form secondary to the decompression of the portal venous system into the systemic circulation. GE varices begin to occur at a pressure gradient of 8 to 10 mm Hg, with bleeding risk increased at a gradient of 12 mm Hg.[7] Esophageal varices are due to dilation of the coronary vein, whereas gastric varices are secondary to backflow through the short gastric veins. The most common location of bleeding is at the GE junction, as this is where the varices are most superficial and have the thinnest wall. Acute variceal bleeding occurs in 25% to 40% of cirrhotic patients and carries a mortality of 25% to 30%, making it one of the most dreaded complications of portal hypertension.[7] In addition to controlling the bleeding by the mechanisms outlined in the next section, prophylactic antibiotics should be administered to this patient population because this intervention decreases mortality.[8]

Less Common Causes

Less common causes of significant upper GI bleeding include cancer, hemobilia, and aortoduodenal fistulas. Gastric cancer often presents late because of its asymptomatic nature early in the disease. When symptoms do arise, they are vague and consist of early satiety, indigestion, melena, or hematemesis. These symptoms portend advanced disease and poor prognosis. Hemobilia is due to a fistula between the splanchnic circulation and the biliary system. Although it may be secondary to a vascular malformation, more commonly there is an inciting cause such as trauma, liver biopsy, or instrumentation of the biliary tree. Aortoduodenal fistula may be primary (from abdominal aortic aneurysm [AAA] before repair) or secondary (after AAA graft placement). An intermittent herald bleed often precedes exsanguinating hemorrhage; therefore, a high index of suspicion is needed to rule out such an etiology early.

CLINICAL PRESENTATION

The clinical presentation varies based on the underlying cause of the upper GI bleed. Commonly encountered findings in the history, physical examination, and laboratory workup of patients with significant upper GI bleeding are summarized in **Table 1**.

WORKUP AND INITIAL TREATMENT
Initial Resuscitation

- Basic ABC: Airway, Breathing, Circulation
- Ensure patent and protected airway
  - Intubate if needed
- Consider mechanical ventilation
- 2 large-bore, peripheral intravenous lines
  - Can consider large-bore central venous catheter or intraosseous line if rapid transfuser will be needed
- Resuscitate with 1:1:1 of packed red blood cells (PRBCs) to fresh frozen plasma (FFP) to platelets
  - Military experience has shown a benefit of resuscitation with fresh whole blood for trauma patients with severe hemorrhage. Although few data exist beyond the trauma setting, many advocate a similar algorithm in all acutely bleeding patients. A 2012 study by Kobayashi and colleagues[9] evaluated hypovolemic shock resuscitation and concluded that early transfusion of 1 PRBC/1 FFP/1 platelets is associated with improved outcomes in patients requiring massive transfusion.
  - Consider massive transfusion protocol
  - Resuscitate to a target hemoglobin of 7 mg/dL. A recent study by Villanueva and colleagues[10] looked at outcomes of patients with acute upper GI bleeding, comparing a transfusion trigger of 7 mg/dL versus 9 mg/dL. This randomized controlled trial showed that a restrictive strategy (goal 7 mg/dL) significantly improved outcomes in comparison with a liberal strategy. Patients with cirrhosis and Childs class A and B disease had the greatest benefit.[10]
- Consider Sengstaken-Blakemore tube for control of immediately life-threatening upper GI bleeding
  - This temporizing measure has been shown to stop life-threatening bleeding in 80% of patients with acute upper GI bleed secondary to esophageal varices. However, owing to the high rate of serious complications (14%) and the high risk of rebleeding once deflated (50%),[7] the Sengstaken-Blakemore tube should be considered a last resort for immediately life-threatening bleeding as a bridge to definitive treatment.

Medical Management

Proton-pump inhibitors
Infusions of proton-pump inhibitors (PPIs) are often used when upper GI bleeding is suspected. The activation of pepsin via gastric acid inhibits platelet aggregation and

Table 1
Clinical presentation of upper GI bleeding

	History	Physical Examination	Laboratory Results
Peptic ulcer disease	Dyspepsia, early satiety, NSAID/ASA use, previous ulcer disease	Hematemesis, possible hematochezia or melena, hemodynamic instability (tachycardia, hypotension)	Decreased hemoglobin, possible increased creatinine, possible increased WBCs, may be *Helicobacter pylori* positive
Mallory-Weiss tear	Vomiting/retching, weakness, dizziness	Hematemesis, possible hematochezia or melena, hemodynamic instability (tachycardia, hypotension)	Decreased hemoglobin, possible increased creatinine, possible increased WBCs
Stress gastritis	History of head injury, severe burns, trauma, mechanical intubation, chronic steroid use, coagulopathy	Hematemesis (coffee grounds more common), melena (slow bleed), not often brisk enough to cause hemodynamic instability	Decreased hemoglobin, increased WBCs
Dieulafoy lesion	Dyspepsia, weakness, dizziness, syncope, or may have no prior history before bleed	Hematemesis (bright red), hematochezia or melena, hemodynamic instability	Decreased hemoglobin, possible decreased hematocrit, Possible increased WBCs
Gastroesophageal varices	Alcohol/tobacco use, Weakness, dizziness, syncope	Stigmata of chronic liver disease, hematemesis, hematochezia or melena, hemodynamic instability	Decreased hemoglobin, possible decreased hematocrit, electrolyte abnormalities, increased bilirubin/liver enzymes
Gastric cancer	Alcohol/tobacco use, often asymptomatic	Hematemesis, melena, palpable supraclavicular or anterior axillary lymph node (late), palpable firm stomach (late)	Decreased hemoglobin, poor nutritional labs, may have elevated CEA or CA 19-9
Hemobilia	Recent trauma, biliary tree instrumentation, gallstones	RUQ abdominal pain, jaundice, hematemesis, melena	Decreased hemoglobin, increased bilirubin, may have increased WBCs
Aortoduodenal fistula	Abdominal pain, back pain, history of AAA repair, may be asymptomatic	Hematemesis or melena (herald bleed), pulsatile abdominal mass	Decreased hemoglobin, may have increased WBCs

Abbreviations: AAA, abdominal aortic aneurysm; ASA, acetylsalicylic acid; CA, cancer antigen; CEA, carcinoembryonic antigen; NSAID, nonsteroidal anti-inflammatory drug; RUQ, right upper quadrant; WBCs, white blood cells.

facilitates clot lysis. When used in high-risk patients, PPI drips reduce the rates of rebleeding, surgery, and mortality.[11]

Octreotide

Octreotide (somatostatin) is an endogenous peptide that reduces splanchnic, hepatic, and azygous blood flow indirectly by inhibiting the vasodilatory effects of glucagon. It is via this mechanism that octreotide is effective at reducing the severity of acute upper GI bleeding secondary to varices. Vasopressin was traditionally the drug of choice for acute variceal bleeding, but it has fallen out of favor since studies have shown somatostatin to have fewer adverse effects and better bleeding control.[12] Though initially used for bleeding control secondary to varices, additional studies have shown somatostatin to be useful for nonvariceal bleeding.[13] However, in the absence of direct comparison with PPIs, they remain second-line medical therapy for this purpose.[14]

Propranolol

Propranolol, a nonselective β-blocker, reduces the hepatic venous pressure gradient and is, therefore, useful in prophylaxis against initial variceal hemorrhage as well as for prevention of recurrent bleeding. Studies have shown a reduction in deaths by 20%.[15] The addition of a nitrate to propranolol increases the chance of the success of medical treatment for acute variceal bleeding, and may be more successful than endoscopic banding in preventing recurrent bleeding.[16]

Tranexamic acid

Tranexamic acid (TXA) is an antifibrinolytic agent that reduces the degradation of fibrin by slowing the conversion of plasminogen to plasmin, thereby supporting clot formation. A Cochrane Library meta-analysis published in 2012 evaluated the utility of TXA versus placebo and versus cimetidine or lansoprazole for upper GI bleeding. Although there was no difference seen in bleeding rates for TXA versus placebo, there was a mortality benefit noted. However, this benefit was not seen when TXA was compared with cimetidine or lansoprazole.[17] While additional evidence is needed before definite treatment recommendations can be made, TXA should be considered part of the armamentarium in severe upper GI hemorrhage (**Fig. 3**).

DEFINITIVE MANAGEMENT
Endoscopy

Endoscopy is a crucial step in both diagnosis of and therapy for upper GI bleeding. Endoscopy can classify the nature of the disease process and provide intervention to stop the bleeding. Early endoscopy should be undertaken (within 24 hours), as early intervention is associated with reduced transfusion needs and a decreased length of stay in high-risk patients with nonvariceal bleeding.[18] In ulcer disease, the presence of either a visible vessel or active bleeding has a high rebleeding rate, with a high need for surgery and an associated mortality of 11%. There is also a potential mortality benefit to early endoscopy, as noted in a retrospective review by Yavorski and colleagues.[19] Various endoscopic interventions are available, and option selected depends on the specific abnormality identified. These interventions commonly include epinephrine injection, thrombin injection, and/or thermocoagulation for ulcers or Dieulafoy lesions. For variceal bleeding, therapeutic options include banding, endoclips, sclerosants, and thrombin injection. If epinephrine is used, the addition of a second endoscopic treatment reduces the incidence of further bleeding, decreases the need for surgery, and has a mortality benefit in patients with high-risk bleeding peptic ulcers.[20] Aside from assessing the mucosa visually, endoscopy also allows for biopsy of suspicious lesions to evaluate for cancer, in addition to diagnosing H pylori infection.

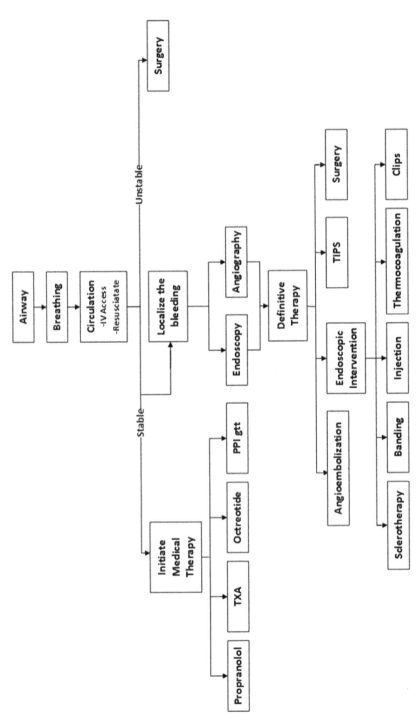

Fig. 3. Decision tree for workup and treatment of upper GI bleeding.

Angioembolization

This radiologic technique is now considered second-line treatment (before surgery) in the 5% to 10% of patients who are unresponsive to medical and endoscopic treatment.[21] Bleeding should be localized by selective catheterization of the most likely artery involved. In the case of upper GI bleeding, the celiac artery should be investigated first, followed by the SMA to evaluate the inferior pancreaticoduodenal artery. If extravasation is noted, superselective embolization (ie, coils, glue, and so forth) is the treatment of choice.[22]

Transjugular Intrahepatic Portosystemic Shunt

Transjugular intrahepatic portosystemic shunt (TIPS) is a minimally invasive way to decompress the portal venous system in patients with portal hypertension. Performed by interventional radiologists, this procedure connects the hepatic vein with the portal vein. This nonselective shunt reduces the rate of rebleeding; however, it does not improve overall survival and has an increased rate of encephalopathy.[23] Complications of TIPS include shunt thrombosis and stenosis, and it may lead to the need for repeated interventions. Therefore, TIPS should be considered for patients with variceal bleeding secondary to portal hypertension only after medical and endoscopic therapy has failed.[7]

Surgical Intervention

In hemodynamically unstable patients secondary to upper GI bleeding that is refractory to resuscitation, primary operative intervention is appropriate, especially if angiography is not immediately available. In addition, surgical intervention may be needed in patients who fail the previously discussed management options.

Table 2	
Surgical options for upper GI bleeding	
Disease Process	**Surgical Options**
Peptic ulcer	Oversew
	3-point ligation of gastroduodenal artery
	Vagotomy and pyloroplasty
	Vagotomy and antrectomy
	Highly selective vagotomy
Mallory-Weiss tear	Oversew
Dieulafoy lesion	Oversew
	Wedge resection
Varices	Portacaval shunt
	Mesocaval shunt
	Distal splenorenal shunt
Gastric cancer	Distal gastrectomy
	Total gastrectomy
	D2 lymphadenectomy
Hemobilia	Selective ligation
	Resection of aneurysm
	Nonselective ligation
	Liver resection
Aortoduodenal fistula	Angiography and stent (if hemodynamically stable)
	Open repair
	Extra-anatomic bypass

Transfusion cutoffs vary, and clinical judgment should supersede a predefined transfusion amount when deciding which patients require surgery. The mortality rate for patients requiring surgery for upper GI bleeding has remained constant over the last decade, likely because of the negative selection of patients after failure of conservative treatment in addition to the increased age and comorbidities of the patient population.[24] Should surgery be required, the procedure of choice depends on the underlying pathophysiology (**Table 2**).

SUMMARY

Upper GI bleeding is still associated with significant morbidity and mortality. The cornerstone of management is initial stabilization, followed by localization and treatment of the bleeding. Medical management and minimally invasive treatments are used primarily and are often successful. Surgery is reserved for patients who fail conservative management.

REFERENCES

1. Sung JJ, Tsoi KK, Ma TK, et al. Causes of mortality in patients with peptic ulcer bleeding: a prospective cohort study of 10,428 cases. Am J Gastroenterol 2010;105(1):84–9.
2. Pilotto A, Maggi S, Noale M, et al. Development and validation of a new questionnaire for the evaluation of upper gastrointestinal symptoms in the elderly population: a multicenter study. J Gerontol A Biol Sci Med Sci 2010;65(2):174–8.
3. Sugawa C, Benishek D, Walt AJ. Mallory-Weiss syndrome. A study of 224 patients. Am J Surg 1983;145(1):30–3.
4. Mallory GK, Weiss SW. Hemorrhages from lacerations of the cardiac orifice of the stomach due to vomiting. Am J Med Sci 1929;178:506–12.
5. Yardley JH, Hendrix TR. Textbook of gastroenterology. 2nd edition. Philadelphia: JB Lippincott Co; 2001. p. 1456–93.
6. Baxter M, Aly EH. Dieulafoy's lesion: current trends in diagnosis and management. Ann R Coll Surg Engl 2010;97(2):548–54.
7. Wright AS, Rikkers LF. Current management of portal hypertension. J Gastrointest Surg 2008;9(5):992–1005.
8. Soares-Weiser K, Brezis M, Tur-Kaspa R, et al. Antibiotic prophylaxis of bacterial infections in cirrhotic inpatients: a meta-analysis of randomized controlled trials. Scand J Gastroenterol 2003;38:193–200.
9. Kobayashi L, Costantini TW, Coimbra R. Hypovolemic shock resuscitation. Surg Clin North Am 2012;92:1403–23.
10. Villanueva C, Colomo A, Bosch A, et al. Transfusion strategies for acute upper gastrointestinal bleeding. N Engl J Med 2013;368(1):11–21.
11. Greenspoon J, Barkun A, Bardou M, et al. Management of patients with nonvariceal upper gastrointestinal bleeding. Clin Gastroenterol Hepatol 2012;10(3):234–9.
12. Imperiale TF, Teran JC, McCullough AJ. A meta-analysis of somatostatin versus vasopressin in the management of acute esophageal variceal hemorrhage. Gastroenterology 1995;109:1289–94.
13. Imperiale TF, Birgisson S. Somatostatin or octreotide compared with H2 antagonists and placebo in the management of acute nonvariceal upper gastrointestinal hemorrhage: a meta-analysis. Ann Intern Med 1997;127(12):1062–71.
14. Wu JC, Sung JJ. Pharmacologic therapy for nonvariceal upper gastrointestinal bleeding. Gastrointest Endosc Clin N Am 2011;21(4):671–9.

15. Hayes PC, Davis JM, Lewis JA, et al. Meta-analysis of value of propranolol in prevention of variceal haemorrhage. Lancet 1990;336:153–6.
16. Villanueva C, Miñana J, Ortiz J, et al. Endoscopic ligation compared with combined treatment with nadolol and isosorbide mononitrate to prevent recurrent variceal bleeding. N Engl J Med 2001;345:647–55.
17. Gluud LL, Klingenberg SL, Langholz E. Tranexamic acid for upper gastrointestinal bleeding (review). Cochrane Database Syst Rev 2012;(1):CD006640.
18. Barkun AN, Bardou M, Kuipers EJ, et al. International consensus recommendations on the management of patients with nonvariceal upper gastrointestinal bleeding. Ann Intern Med 2010;152(2):101–13.
19. Yavorski RT, Wong RK, Maydonovitch C, et al. Analysis of 3,294 cases of upper gastrointestinal bleeding in military medical facilities. Am J Gastroenterol 1995; 90(4):568–73.
20. Calvet X, Vergara M, Brullet E, et al. Addition of a second endoscopic treatment following epinephrine injection improves outcome in high-risk bleeding ulcers. Gastroenterology 2004;126(2):441–50.
21. Loffroy R, Rao P, Ota S, et al. Embolization of acute nonvariceal upper gastrointestinal hemorrhage resistant to endoscopic treatment: results and predictors of recurrent bleeding. Cardiovasc Intervent Radiol 2010;33(6):1088–100.
22. Walker TG, Salazar GM, Waltman AC. Angiographic evaluation and management of acute gastrointestinal hemorrhage. World J Gastroenterol 2012;18(11):1191–201.
23. Papatheodoridis GV, Goulis J, Leandro G, et al. Transjugular intrahepatic portosystemic shunt compared with endoscopic treatment for prevention of variceal rebleeding: a meta-analysis. Hepatology 1999;30:612–22.
24. Czymek R, Großmann A, Roblick U, et al. Surgical management of acute upper gastrointestinal bleeding: still a major challenge. Hepatogastroenterology 2012; 59(115):768–73.

Lower Gastrointestinal Bleeding

Marcie Feinman, MD, Elliott R. Haut, MD*

KEYWORDS

- Hematochezia • Melena • Diverticulosis • Angiodysplasia

KEY POINTS

- Lower gastrointestinal bleeding is likely under-reported and remains a common causes of emergency department visits.
- Localization of bleeding is key to forming an appropriate treatment plan.
- Whether the bleeding is occult, moderate, or severe dictates the workup.
- Hemodynamically unstable patients require immediate intervention.
- Although minimally invasive techniques are often sufficient to stop the bleeding, there is still a role for surgery in certain patient populations.

INTRODUCTION

Lower gastrointestinal (GI) bleeding has an annual incidence of about 20 to 27 cases per 100,000 population in developed countries. However, it is thought that this number is falsely low because of the substantial number of patients who do not seek medical care.[1] Although lower GI bleeding is not as common as upper GI bleeding, it remains a frequent cause of hospital admissions and carries a mortality of up to 10% to 20%.

Lower GI bleeding can be classified into 3 groups based on the severity of bleeding: occult lower GI bleeding, moderate lower GI bleeding, and severe lower GI bleeding.

Patients of any age can present with occult lower GI bleeding. Because the bleed tends to be slow and chronic, patients have microcytic, hypochromic anemia. Stool guiac will be positive.

Often presenting with melena or hematochezia, moderate bleeding can occur in patients of any age. Despite the obvious bleeding, patients remain hemodynamically stable.

Patients with severe lower GI bleeding present hemodynamically unstable with heart rates greater than 100 and systolic blood pressure less than 90. They have associated low urine output and decreased hemoglobin levels. Hematochezia is

Division of Acute Care Surgery, Department of Surgery, Anesthesiology/Critical Care Medicine (ACCM), Emergency Medicine, The Johns Hopkins University School of Medicine, Sheikh Zayed Tower, 1800 Orleans Street, Suite 6017, Baltimore, MD 21287, USA
* Corresponding author.
E-mail address: ehaut1@jhmi.edu

Surg Clin N Am 94 (2014) 55–63
http://dx.doi.org/10.1016/j.suc.2013.10.005
0039-6109/14/$ – see front matter © 2014 Elsevier Inc. All rights reserved.

prominent. This tends to occur in elderly patients older than 65 years and has an associated mortality of 21%.[2]

BLOOD SUPPLY

Lower GI bleeding is defined as any bleed that occurs distal to the ligament of Treitz. Although the colon is the most likely source of bleeding, small bowel disease can occur. In addition, upper GI sources must always be considered in a patient who presents with bleeding per rectum.

Midgut

The midgut is defined as all structures between the foregut and the hindgut. This includes the distal duodenum, jejunum, ileum, appendix, cecum, ascending colon, hepatic flexure, and proximal transverse colon. The superior mesenteric artery (SMA) and its branches provide the blood supply to the midgut. Venous drainage is via the portal system.

Hindgut

The hindgut includes the distal one-third of the transverse colon, the splenic flexure, descending colon, sigmoid colon, and rectum. Blood supply is mainly via the inferior mesenteric artery (IMA), with rectal perfusion through the superior, middle, and inferior rectal arteries. Venous drainage is via the portal system, with the exception of the lower rectum, which drains into the systemic circulation.

The SMA and IMA are connected by the marginal artery of Drummond. This vascular arcade runs in the mesentery close to the bowel and is almost always present. As patients age, there is increased incidence of occlusion of the IMA. The left colon stays perfused, primarily because of the marginal artery (**Fig. 1**).

PATHOPHYSIOLOGY

Lower GI bleeding has multiple causes, each with its own morbidity attributed to the underlying pathophysiology. Multiple studies of the incidence and etiology of lower GI bleeding found that diverticulosis was the most common at 30%, followed by anorectal disease (14%–20%), ischemia (12%), inflammatory bowel disease (IBD) (9%), neoplasia (6%) and arteriovenous (AV) malformations (3%).[3,4]

Diverticulosis

With age, the colonic wall weakens and develops diverticula. These saclike protrusions generally occur where the penetrating vessel perforates through the circular muscle fibers, resulting in only mucosa separating the vessel from the bowel lumen. It is estimated that approximately 50% of adults over the age of 60 have radiologic evidence of diverticula, most commonly in the descending and sigmoid colon, and 20% of these patients will go on to develop bleeding. Despite the majority of diverticula being on the left side of the colon, diverticular bleeding originates from the right side of the colon in 50% to 90% of instances.[5] This bleeding stops spontaneously in the most patients; however, in about 5% of patients, the bleeding can be massive and life-threatening.

Anorectal Disease

Anorectal disease encompasses many etiologies, including hemorrhoids and anal fissures.

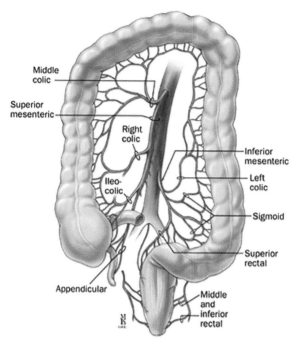

Fig. 1. Arterial blood supply of the colon and rectum. (*Courtesy of* Johns Hopkins Medicine Colorectal Center, Baltimore, MD. Available at: http://www.hopkinscoloncancercenter.org/CMS/CMS_Page.aspx?CurrentUDV=59&CMS_Page_ID=1F7C07D4-268D-4635-8975-70A594870CC8.)

Hemorrhoids

Hemorrhoids may be internal or external, although internal hemorrhoids (above the dentate line) are generally the type that cause rapid rectal bleeding. Hemorrhoids are engorged vessels in the normal anal cushions. When swollen, this tissue is very friable and susceptible to trauma, which leads to painless, bright red bleeding.

Anal fissures

Fissures begin with a tear in the anal mucosa. The tear may resolve, in which case it is an acute anal fissure, or it may persist and become a chronic anal fissure. With the passage of stool, the mucosa continues to tear and leads to bright red bleeding. Anal fissures generally occur in the midline, and any fissure off the midline should prompt a workup for an underlying etiology.

Mesenteric Ischemia

Mesenteric ischemia is caused by a mismatch in the supply and demand of oxygen at the level of the small intestine. Most commonly, this is caused by inadequate circulation to the bowel and may be embolic, thombotic, or nonocclusive (NOMI) in nature. For symptoms to occur, 2 or more vessels (celiac, SMA, or IMA) need to be affected. Cardiac disease and known atherosclerosis are big risk factors for acute mesenteric ischemia secondary to emboli or thromboses. NOMI affects critically ill patients who are vasopressor dependent. The vasoconstriction caused by these medications (especially vasopressin) results in a low-flow state to the small bowel.[6] Venous thrombosis of the visceral vessels can also precipitate an acute ischemic event.

Compromised venous return leads to interstitial swelling in the bowel wall, with subsequent impedance of arterial flow and eventual necrosis.

Ischemic Colitis

Ischemic colitis is caused by poor perfusion of the colon, which results in the inability of that area of the colon to meet its metabolic demands. It can be gangrenous or nongangrenous, acute, transient, or chronic. The left colon is predominantly affected, with the splenic flexure having increased susceptibility.[7] Intraluminal hemorrhage occurs as the mucosa becomes necrotic, sloughs, and bleeds. Damage to the tissue is caused both with the ischemic insult as well as reperfusion injury. The colon is affected from the mucosa outward, with perforation a late finding only after all layers of the colon are involved.

Inflammatory Bowel Disease

Crohn disease and ulcerative colitis are the main disease states under the heading of IBD. Both are autoimmune in nature and lead to unopposed inflammation.

Crohn disease

T cell activation stimulates interleukin (IL)-12 and tumor necrosis factor (TNF)-α, which causes chronic inflammation and tissue injury. Initially, inflammation starts focally around the crypts, followed by superficial ulceration of the mucosa. The deep mucosal layers are then invaded in a noncontinuous fashion, and noncaseating granulomas form, which can invade through the entire thickness of the bowel and into the mesentery and surrounding structures.[8] The granulomas are pathognomonic of Crohn disease; however, their absence does not exclude this diagnosis.

Ulcerative colitis

T cells cytotoxic to the colonic epithelium accumulate in the lamina propria, accompanied by B cells that secrete immunoglobulin G (IgG) and IgE. This results in inflammation of the crypts of Lieberkuhn, with abscesses and pseudopolyps.[8] Whereas Crohn disease can affect any part of the GI tract, ulcerative colitis generally begins at the rectum and is a continuous process confined exclusively to the colon.

Neoplasia

Colon carcinoma follows a distinct progression from polyp to cancer. Mutations of multiple genes are required for the formation of adenocarcinoma, including the APC gene, Kras, DCC, and p53. Certain hereditary syndromes are also classified by defects in DNA mismatch repair genes and microsatellite instability. These tumors tend to bleed slowly, and patients present with hemocult positive stools and microcytic anemia. Although cancers of the small bowel are much less common than colorectal cancers, they should be ruled out in cases of lower GI bleeding in which no other source is identified.

AV Malformation/Angiodysplasia

AV malformation

These direct connections between arteries and veins can occur in the colonic submucosa (or anywhere else in the GI tract). The lack of capillary buffers causes high pressure blood to enter directly into the venous system, making these vessels at high risk of rupture into the bowel lumen.

Angiodysplasia

Over time, previously healthy blood vessels of the cecum and ascending colon degenerate and become prone to bleeding. Although 75% of angiodysplasia cases involve the right colon, they are a significant cause of obscure bleeding and the most common cause of bleeding from the small bowel in the elderly.[9]

CLINICAL PRESENTATION

Lower GI bleeding can range from occult to massive and life threatening. The clinical findings differ based on the severity of the bleed and the underlying cause. **Table 1** consists of possible signs/symptoms/laboratory values with which patients with lower GI bleeding may present. Some things do not help figure out source—weakness, dizziness, syncope.

WORKUP AND INITIAL TREATMENT

Workup should begin with resuscitation as needed (covered more fully in the upper GI section).

Next, one should rule out an upper GI source of bleeding. Nasogastric tube (NGT) lavage should be performed in all patients with lower GI bleeding to rule out an upper GI source. In order to completely exclude an upper GI bleed, the NGT lavage must return bilious fluid without blood. Obtaining clear fluid only, while favoring a lower GI source, does not completely rule out duodenal bleeding distal to the pylorus, but proximal to the ligament of Treitz (classically a duodenal ulcer).

LOCALIZE AND STOP THE BLEEDING

Many options exist to determine where the bleeding originates from when distal to the ligament of Treitz. Which test or combination of tests to choose is determined by the patient's age, medical history, rate of bleeding, and hemodynamic stability.

Colonoscopy

Often considered the initial diagnostic modality of choice, colonoscopy can identify the origin of severe LGI bleeding in 74% to 82% of patients.[10] This invasive procedure is not without disadvantages. In order to be effective, a mechanical bowel preparation is sometimes performed, which will delay the endoscopy. A mechanical bowel preparation is not required, especially in those patients with rapid bleeding, because the blood will often act as cathartic to clean out the colon. In addition, patients require sedation, which carries its own risks. As long as patients remain stable during the bowel preparation and sedation, colonoscopy then has the advantage of not only localizing the source of bleeding, but also allowing intervention via clips, epinephrine injection, thermoregulation, or laser photocoagulation. Per the Scottish Intercollegiate Guidelines Network (SIGN) guidelines, in patients with massive lower GI bleeding, colonoscopic hemostasis is an effective means of controlling bleeding from a diverticular source when appropriately skilled providers are available.[11] Studies have looked into the timing of colonoscopy to attempt to ascertain if early endoscopy has any benefit. A randomized, controlled trial found that urgent colonoscopy (defined as within 8 hours of presentation) had improved diagnosis but not improved outcomes as compared to standard colonoscopy (within 48 hours of presentation).[12]

Table 1
Clinical presentation of lower GI bleeding

	History	Physical Examination	Laboratory Findings
Diverticulosis	Can have bloating or cramping, afebrile, often symptomatic	Hematochezia (brisk bleed/left colon) or melena (slow bleed/right colon), no abdominal tenderness	Decreased hemoglobin, possible microcytic hypochromic anemia (chronic occult bleed)
Crohn disease	Crampy abdominal pain, diarrhea, steatorrhea, fatigue, weight loss, arthritis, eye complaints, skin disorders, renal stones	Stool guiac positive, abdominal tenderness, possible right lower quadrant mass, possible enterocutaneous fistula, possible anal fissure/fistula	Microcytic hypochromic anemia, B12 deficiency, elevated C-reactive protein (CRP)/erythrocyte sedimentation rate (ESR), increased white blood cells (WBCs)
Ulcerative colitis	Colicky abdominal pain, urgency, tenesmus, incontinence, diarrhea or constipation (if distal disease)	Gross blood on rectal examination, abdominal tenderness, peripheral edema, muscle wasting	Anemia, elevated ESR, low albumin, elevated fecal lactoferrin, possible elevated alkaline phosphatase
Mesenteric ischemia	Pain out of proportion to examination (periumbilical), nausea/vomiting, bloody diarrhea, weight loss, food avoidance	Minimal findings, no peritonitis, stool guiac positive	Increased WBCs, increased lactate, metabolic acidosis, possible elevated amylase
Ischemic colitis	Mild-to-moderate abdominal pain (lateral), bloody diarrhea	Abdominal tenderness (left greater than right), gross blood on rectal examination	Increased WBCs, elevated lactate, amylase, creatine phosphokinase (CPK) and lactate dehydrogenase (LDH), metabolic acidosis, anemia
Hemorrhoids	Painless bleeding, itching, mild incontinence, history of cirrhosis	Prolapsed hemorrhoids, gross blood on rectal examination, stigmata of liver disease	Iron deficiency anemia (if chronic), possible elevated liver function tests/coagulopathy
Anal fissure	Tearing pain with bowel movements, perianal pruritis	Severe pain on rectal examination, bright red blood	Often normal
Neoplasia	Abdominal pain, distention, decreased caliber of stool, tenesmus, rectal pain, weight loss	Palpable mass, abdominal tenderness, guiac-positive stool, rectal mass on direct rectal examination (DRE), pallor	Microcytic hypochromic anemia, possible elevated carcinoembryonic antigen
AV malformation/angiodysplasia	Painless rectal bleeding	Asymptomatic, hematochezia, or melena	Anemia

Nuclear Scintigraphy

This diagnostic modality can detect bleeding rates between 0.1 and 0.5 cc/min. Considered 10 times more sensitive than mesenteric angiography for detecting bleeding, nuclear scintigraphy is a sensitive diagnostic tool (86% sensitivity). However, the specificity is only 50%. One study by Ng and colleagues[13] determined that time to positivity of a nuclear medicine scan helped guide further treatment. If a blush was seen within 2 minutes of starting the scan, there was a positive predictive value of 75% on angiography. Conversely, if the blush occurred beyond 2 minutes, this was associated with a negative predictive value of 93% for angiography. In addition to low specificity, nuclear scintigraphy has several other disadvantages. These include the lack of ability to intervene during the study, as well as the fact that patients need to be actively bleeding at the time of the test to have a positive result. Because of this, many authors advocate using nuclear scintigraphy as a screening modality only to determine which patients would benefit from mesenteric angiography. While not a strong recommendation, the SIGN guidelines suggest considering nuclear scintigraphy to assist in localizing lower GI bleeding in patients with recent hemorrhage.[11]

Angiography

Angiography can be used when colonoscopy fails to localize a bleeding source, or when bleeding is so brisk as to preclude colonoscopy as a useful diagnostic modality. Requiring a minimum bleed of 0.5 cc/min, angiography has the benefit of being both diagnostic and potentially therapeutic in brisk bleeds. Interventions include selective vasopressin infusions and superselective angioembolization. Generally, the SMA is investigated first, because much lower GI bleeding arises from the right colon. This is followed by the IMA next and the celiac trunk last, if necessary. The disadvantages of angiography include a low sensitivity (only about 30%–47%) and the requirement of a substantial amount of active bleeding at the time of the study in order to be positive. However, if the patient does have brisk active bleeding, emergency angiography and vasopressin infusion have been shown to improve operative morbidity, mortality, and outcome.[14] In patients with massive lower GI bleeding, if colonoscopy fails to identify and control the site of hemorrhage, transarterial embolization is recommended.[11]

Surgical Intervention

Emergency surgery may be needed to control bleeding in about 10% to 25% of patients in whom nonoperative management is unsuccessful or unavailable.[15] Indications for emergent surgery include hemodynamic instability with active bleeding, persistent recurrent bleeding, or transfusion requirement of greater than 6 units of packed red blood cells (PRBCs) in 24 hours with active bleeding.[10] Patients requiring ten or more units of PRBCs in 24 hours have a significantly greater mortality than patients who receive less than 10 units of blood (45% vs 7%).[16] Therefore, the commonly accepted transfusion trigger to perform surgery for a lower GI bleed is 6 units of PRBCs to avoid the mortality associated with giving more blood and delaying definitive management. If emergency surgery is required, definitive localization of the bleeding site is ideal, because segmental colonic resection is preferred. However, segmental resection should be avoided unless the source is definitely identified, because this operation is associated with high rebleeding, morbidity, and mortality rates. If the bleed cannot be localized, a subtotal colectomy is the recommended procedure. Bleeding caused by tumors should be resected with the appropriate oncologic procedure to ensure adequate margins and lymph nodes in the specimen.

OBSCURE BLEEDING

Although the colon is by far the most likely source of lower GI bleeding, the small bowel can also be affected. This part of the GI tract has traditionally been difficult to evaluate; however, many new modalities are available for visualization. Wireless capsule endoscopy is the most widely used for diagnosis of small bowel bleeding. Although it does not have therapeutic capabilities, capsule endoscopy is noninvasive and allows visualization of the complete small bowel, leading to improved diagnosis over alternative modalities.[17] Other options for diagnosis of a small bowel source of bleeding are push enteroscopy or double balloon enteroscopy. Despite the potential therapeutic advantage of enteroscopy, the invasive nature of the procedure and the ability to only evaluate the most proximal 60 cm of jejunum make these options less attractive than capsule endoscopy. Surgical management of massive occult lower GI bleeding may include the use of intraoperative enteroscopy. Intraoperative Enteroscopy (IOE) remains indicated when: (1) small bowel lesions have been identified by a preoperative work-up; (2) lesions cannot be managed by angio-embolization and/or endoscopic methods, or when surgery is required for complete treatment (ie, small bowel tumors), and (3) bleeding cannot be localized during surgical explorations. The ability of IOE to identify bleeding lesions is good and has been shown to be equal to the video capsule endoscopy diagnostic yield, with a higher sensitivity than push–pull enteroscopy.[18] However, this invasive procedure carries a 16.8% morbidity and should only be used if all other methods fail.[19]

SUMMARY

Although not as common as upper GI bleeding, bleeding that originates distal to the ligament of Treitz remains a frequent cause of hospital admissions, with a significant associated morbidity and mortality. Workup should focus on stabilization of the patient primarily, followed by localization and cessation of the bleed. Various modalities exist for these purposes and should be chosen based on patient presentation and severity of the bleeding. Although incredible advances have been made in minimally invasive options for treatment of lower GI bleeds, surgery remains a viable option for patients who remain unstable despite adequate resuscitation and for those who fail more conservative treatments.

REFERENCES

1. Talley NJ, Jones M. Self-reported rectal bleeding in a United States community: prevalence, risk factors, and health care seeking. Am J Gastroenterol 1998; 93(11):2179–83.
2. Longstreth GF. Epidemiology and outcome of patients hospitalized with acute lower gastrointestinal hemorrhage: a population-based study. Am J Gastroenterol 1997;92(3):419–24.
3. Ghassemi KA, Jensen DM. Lower GI bleeding: epidemiology and management. Curr Gastroenterol Rep 2013;15:333.
4. Gayer C, Chino A, Lucas C, et al. Acute lower gastrointestinal bleeding in 1,112 patients admitted to an urban emergency medical center. Surgery 2009;146(4): 600–6 [discussion: 606–7].
5. Meyers MA, Alonso DR, Gray GF, et al. Pathogenesis of bleeding colonic diverticulosis. Gastroenterology 1976;71(4):577–83.
6. Chang RW, Chang JB, Longo W. Update in management of mesenteric ischemia. World J Gastroenterol 2006;12(20):3243–7.

7. Theodoropoulou A, Koutroubakis IE. Ischemic colitis: clinical practice in diagnosis and treatment. World J Gastroenterol 2008;14(48):7302–8.
8. Thoreson R, Cullen JJ. Pathophysiology of inflammatory bowel disease: an overview. Surg Clin North Am 2007;87(3):575–85.
9. Regula J, Wronska E, Pachlewski J. Vascular lesions of the gastrointestinal tract. Best Pract Res Clin Gastroenterol 2008;22(2):313–28.
10. Vernava AM III, Moore BA, Longo WE, et al. Lower gastrointestinal bleeding. Dis Colon Rectum 1997;40(7):846–58.
11. Scottish Intercollegiate Guidelines Network (SIGN). Management of acute upper and lower gastrointestinal bleeding. A national clinical guideline. SIGN Publication; no. 105. Edinburgh (Scotland): Scottish Intercollegiate Guidelines Network (SIGN); 2008.
12. Green BT, Rockey DC, Portwood G, et al. Urgent colonoscopy for evaluation and management of acute lower gastrointestinal hemorrhage: a randomized controlled trial. Am J Gastroenterol 2005;100(11):2395–402.
13. Ng DA, Opelka FG, Beck DE, et al. Predictive value of technetium Tc 99m-labeled red blood cell scintigraphy for positive angiogram in massive lower gastrointestinal hemorrhage. Dis Colon Rectum 1997;40(4):471–7.
14. Browder W, Cerise EJ, Litwin MS. Impact of emergency angiography in massive lower gastrointestinal bleeding. Ann Surg 1986;204(5):530–6.
15. Chalasani N, Wilcox CM. Etiology and outcome of lower gastrointestinal bleeding in patients with AIDS. Am J Gastroenterol 1998;93(2):175–8.
16. Bender JS, Wiencek RG, Bouwman DL. Morbidity and mortality following total abdominal colectomy for massive lower gastrointestinal bleeding. Am Surg 1991;57:536–41.
17. Ell C, Remke S, May A, et al. The first prospective controlled trial comparing wireless capsule endoscopy with push enteroscopy in chronic gastrointestinal bleeding. Endoscopy 2002;34(9):685–9.
18. Hartmann D, Schmidt H, Bolz G, et al. A prospective two-center study comparing wireless capsule endoscopy with intraoperative enteroscopy in patients with obscure GI bleeding. Gastrointest Endosc 2005;61:826–32.
19. Bonnet S, Douard R, Malamut G, et al. Intraoperative enteroscopy in the management of obscure gastrointestinal bleeding. Dig Liver Dis 2013;45(4):277–84.

Spontaneous Hemoperitoneum

George Kasotakis, MD, MPH

KEYWORDS

- Spontaneous hemoperitoneum • Rupture • Agioembolization

KEY POINTS

- Spontaneous hemoperitoneum is a rare, but life-threatening condition usually caused by nontraumatic rupture of the liver, spleen, or abdominal vasculature with underlying pathology.
- Management revolves around angioembolization or surgical intervention.
- It is typically seen in anticoagulated or coagulopathic patients and may prove rapidly fatal, if not managed appropriately.

Spontaneous hemoperitoneum (SH) is a rare, but life-threatening condition that is defined as blood within the peritoneal cavity of nontraumatic etiology.[1,2] Given the rarity of SH, its diagnosis is almost always unsuspected until the time of imaging, which is undertaken in patients who present with acute abdominal pain and/or distention and anemia. Implicit in making this diagnosis is a nontraumatic cause, and high quality imaging is of paramount importance in identifying the underlying cause.

SH most commonly arises from hepatic, splenic, vascular or gynecologic pathology (the latter will not be discussed here, as it is outside the scope of this text), and usually in anticoagulated or coagulopathic subjects (**Box 1**).[3,4] It requires the emergent attention of the treating clinician, as it can prove rapidly fatal, even if managed appropriately. It typically presents with signs of acute intraperitoneal bleeding, namely abdominal pain and distention, tachycardia, and even hypotension and abdominal compartment syndrome in severe cases.

Imaging is essential in cases of nontraumatic hemoperitoneum in that it establishes the diagnosis of SH and helps identify its primary etiology. Although computed tomography (CT) is the most commonly used modality in patients with acute abdominal pain, ultrasound may be used when gynecologic conditions are considered, or, less commonly, if the patient is too unstable to be transferred to the CT suite and the treating clinician is attempting to grossly localize the hemorrhage. CT, however, is superior in that it can point to a specific organ as the source of the bleeding; detect active hemorrhage (active contrast extravasation or blush in contrasted studies); and provide information on how long ago the hemorrhagic episode took place (varying Hounsfield units of fresh, clotted, and lysed blood).[2,5]

Section of Trauma & Acute Care Surgery, Boston Medical Center, Boston University School of Medicine, 840 Harrison Avenue, Dowling 2 South, #2414, Boston, MA 02118, USA
E-mail address: gkasot@bu.edu

Surg Clin N Am 94 (2014) 65–69
http://dx.doi.org/10.1016/j.suc.2013.10.006
0039-6109/14/$ – see front matter © 2014 Elsevier Inc. All rights reserved.
surgical.theclinics.com

Box 1
Nongynecologic causes of spontaneous hemoperitoneum

1. Hepatic

    Benign

        Adenomas

        Focal nodular hyperplasias

        Hemangiomas

        Infiltrative diseases (amyloidosis)

    Malignant

        Primary hepatocellular carcinoma

        Metastatic disease

        Angiosarcomas

    Infiltrative diseases

        Amyloidosis

2. Splenic

    Infections

        Cytomegalovirus

        EBV

        HIV

        Malaria

        Bartonella

    Malignancies

        Lymphomas

        Leukemias

        Angiosarcomas

    Infiltrative diseases

        Amyloidosis

        Gaucher disease

3. Vascular

    Arterial

        Aneurysms

        Pseudoaneurysms

        Mycotic aneurysms

        Dissection

    Venous

        Pelvic veins during labor

        Abdominal varices

LIVER

The liver is considered as the most common cause of SH, when gynecologic causes are not considered, with anticoagulation, pregnancy, and minor (usually unreported) trauma being the most common triggering factors. In most cases, liver masses, typically undiagnosed, rupture spontaneously and present as SH. These can be benign or malignant. The former include hepatic adenomas,[6] focal nodular hyperplasias,[7] large hemangiomas,[8] or rarely infiltrative hepatic diseases such as amyloidosis.[9] Hepatic adenomas are typically seen in pregnant[6] or oral steroid contraceptive-using women,[10] or less commonly in anabolic steroid-taking males.[11] Less frequently, multiple hormone-independent hepatic adenomas may outgrow their vascular supply, necrose, and eventually rupture, leading to SH. Large hemangiomas may also rupture during pregnancy, likely because of the large intravascular volume associated with gestation. Malignant hepatic lesions, either primary or metastatic, may also rupture spontaneously. In fact, hepatocellular carcinoma (HCC) constitutes the most commonly identified pathology in SH arising from the liver,[12] and when nontraumatic hemoperitoneum is seen on CT, HCC should be considered the most likely etiology, especially when an irregular mass is seen within the hepatic parenchyma. Primary hepatic angiosarcomas and metastatic disease are far less frequent causes of SH.[12,13]

SPLEEN

Even though the spleen is the second most common solid organ to give rise to SH, spontaneous splenic rupture (SSR) is exceedingly rare.[14,15] Unlike the liver, SSR is typically not associated with parenchymal masses, but with infectious (most notably cytomegalovirus, Epstein-Barr virus [EBV], human immunodeficiency virus [HIV], malaria, and bartonellosis)[16–21] or inflammatory processes.[22,23] Less commonly, infiltrative diseases (Gaucher disease, splenic amyloidosis)[24,25] or hematologic malignancies (lymphomas, leukemias, angiosarcomas) may be the underlying pathology.[26,27]

VASCULAR CAUSES

Vascular causes of SH include aneurysms, pseudoaneurysms, and mycotic aneurysms or arterial dissection complicated with rupture.[2,28,29] The celiac, superior mesenteric, and renal arteries are most commonly affected,[30] with extensive atherosclerotic disease and vasculitis being the most commonly cited predisposing factors.[31,32] Spontaneous arterial rupture is a catastrophic event, with mortality rates that exceed 30%.[2] Presence of hemoperitoneum on imaging without associated hepatic or splenic pathology typically alerts radiologists to closely evaluate the abdominal vasculature; however, pathology may not always be easily identifiable.

Less commonly, venous rupture may be the cause of SH. Common clinical scenarios include those of rupture of enlarged pelvic veins during labor or abdominal varices that have developed over time secondary to cirrhosis and portal hypertension.[33–35] Contrary to what one might expect, prognosis after spontaneous venous bleeding is much worse compared with that of arterial etiology.

MANAGEMENT

Regardless of the underlying etiology of SH, angiography and embolization almost always constitute first-line therapy in the hemodynamically stable patient. Surgery should be considered in persistently hypotensive patients, or in those in whom interventional techniques have failed to control the bleeding. Options for hemorrhage control during surgery include, but are not limited to, repair (either primary or reinforced with native tissue or biologic prosthetics), partial (or complete in the case of the spleen) resection, electro- and Argon beam coagulation, tissue sealants, local hemostatics, and vascular ligation.[36]

REFERENCES

1. Furlan A, Fakhran S, Federle MP. Spontaneous abdominal hemorrhage: causes, CT findings, and clinical implications. AJR Am J Roentgenol 2009;193(4): 1077–87.
2. Lucey BC, Varghese JC, Anderson SW, et al. Spontaneous hemoperitoneum: a bloody mess. Emerg Radiol 2007;14(2):65–75.
3. Ghobrial MW, Karim M, Mannam S. Spontaneous splenic rupture following the administration of intravenous heparin: case report and retrospective case review. Am J Hematol 2002;71(4):314–7.
4. Moore CH, Snashall J, Boniface K, et al. Spontaneous splenic hemorrhage after initiation of dabigatran (Pradaxa) for atrial fibrillation. Am J Emerg Med 2012; 30(9):2082.e1–2.
5. Mortele KJ, Cantisani V, Brown DL, et al. Spontaneous intraperitoneal hemorrhage: imaging features. Radiol Clin North Am 2003;41(6):1183–201.
6. Estebe JP, Malledant Y, Guillou YM, et al. Spontaneous rupture of an adenoma of the liver during pregnancy. J Chir (Paris) 1988;125(11):654–6.
7. Kleespies A, Settmacher U, Neuhaus P. Spontaneous rupture of hepatic focal nodular hyperplasia—a rare cause of acute intraabdominal bleeding. Zentralbl Chir 2002;127(4):326–8.
8. Corigliano N, Mercantini P, Amodio PM, et al. Hemoperitoneum from a spontaneous rupture of a giant hemangioma of the liver: report of a case. Surg Today 2003;33(6):459–63.
9. Battula N, Tsapralis D, Morgan M, et al. Spontaneous liver haemorrhage and haemobilia as initial presentation of undiagnosed polyarteritis nodosa. Ann R Coll Surg Engl 2012;94(4):e163–5.
10. Khan S, Smulders YM, de Vries JI, et al. Life-threatening complications of hormonal contraceptives: a case history. Case Rep Obstet Gynecol 2013;2013: 186230.
11. Bagia S, Hewitt PM, Morris DL. Anabolic steroid-induced hepatic adenomas with spontaneous haemorrhage in a bodybuilder. Aust N Z J Surg 2000;70(9): 686–7.
12. Chen ZY, Qi QH, Dong ZL. Etiology and management of hemmorrhage in spontaneous liver rupture: a report of 70 cases. World J Gastroenterol 2002;8(6): 1063–6.
13. Burke M, Opeskin K. Spontaneous rupture of the liver associated with a primary angiosarcoma: case report. Am J Forensic Med Pathol 2000;21(2):134–7.
14. Tataria M, Dicker RA, Melcher M, et al. Spontaneous splenic rupture: the masquerade of minor trauma. J Trauma 2005;59(5):1228–30.
15. Amonkar SJ, Kumar EN. Spontaneous rupture of the spleen: three case reports and causative processes for the radiologist to consider. Br J Radiol 2009; 82(978):e111–3.
16. Rinderknecht AS, Pomerantz WJ. Spontaneous splenic rupture in infectious mononucleosis: case report and review of the literature. Pediatr Emerg Care 2012;28(12):1377–9.
17. Vallabhaneni S, Scott H, Carter J, et al. Atraumatic splenic rupture: an unusual manifestation of acute HIV infection. AIDS Patient Care STDS 2011;25(8):461–4.

18. Bellaiche G, Habib E, Baledent F, et al. Hemoperitoneum due to spontaneous splenic rupture: a rare complication of primary cytomegalovirus infection. Gastroenterol Clin Biol 1998;22(1):107–8.
19. Daybell D, Paddock CD, Zaki SR, et al. Disseminated infection with *Bartonella henselae* as a cause of spontaneous splenic rupture. Clin Infect Dis 2004; 39(3):e21–4.
20. Bansal VK, Krishna A, Misra MC, et al. Spontaneous splenic rupture in complicated malaria: non-operative management. Trop Gastroenterol 2010;31(3):233–5.
21. Gockel HR, Heidemann J, Lorenz D, et al. Spontaneous splenic rupture, in tertian malaria. Infection 2006;34(1):43–5.
22. Patel VG, Eltayeb OM, Zakaria M, et al. Spontaneous subcapsular splenic hematoma: a rare complication of pancreatitis. Am Surg 2005;71(12):1066–9.
23. Gandhi V, Philip S, Maydeo A, et al. Ruptured subcapsular giant haematoma of the spleen—a rare complication of acute pancreatitis. Trop Gastroenterol 2010; 31(2):123–4.
24. Khan AZ, Escofet X, Roberts KM, et al. Spontaneous splenic rupture–a rare complication of amyloidosis. Swiss Surg 2003;9(2):92–4.
25. Stone DL, Ginns EI, Krasnewich D, et al. Life-threatening splenic hemorrhage in two patients with Gaucher disease. Am J Hematol 2000;64(2):140–2.
26. Chappuis J, Simoens C, Smets D, et al. Spontaneous rupture of the spleen in relation to a non-Hodgkin lymphoma. Acta Chir Belg 2007;107(4):446–8.
27. Goddard SL, Chesney AE, Reis MD, et al. Pathological splenic rupture: a rare complication of chronic myelomonocytic leukemia. Am J Hematol 2007;82(5): 405–8.
28. Chookun J, Bounes V, Ducasse JL, et al. Rupture of splenic artery aneurysm during early pregnancy: a rare and catastrophic event. Am J Emerg Med 2009; 27(7):898.e5–6.
29. Okada T, Frank M, Pellerin O, et al. Embolization of life-threatening arterial rupture in patients with vascular Ehlers-Danlos syndrome. Cardiovasc Intervent Radiol 2013. [Epub ahead of print].
30. Yoo BR, Han HY, Cho YK, et al. Spontaneous rupture of a middle colic artery aneurysm arising from superior mesenteric artery dissection: diagnosis by color Doppler ultrasonography and CT angiography. J Clin Ultrasound 2012;40(4): 255–9.
31. Obon-Dent M, Shabaneh B, Dougherty KG, et al. Spontaneous celiac artery dissection case report and literature review. Tex Heart Inst J 2012;39(5):703–6.
32. Jia ZZ, Zhao JW, Tian F, et al. Initial and middle-term results of treatment for symptomatic spontaneous isolated dissection of superior mesenteric artery. Eur J Vasc Endovasc Surg 2013;45(5):502–8.
33. Ajmal M. Spontaneous splenic vein bleeding during pregnancy: consequences of a missed diagnosis. J Anesth 2012;26(6):959–60.
34. Leaute F, Frampas E, Mathon G, et al. Massive hemoperitoneum from rupture of an intra-peritoneal varix. J Radiol 2002;83(11):1775–7.
35. Moreno JP, Pina R, Rodriguez F, et al. Spontaneous hemoperitoneum caused by intraabdominal variceal rupture in a patient with liver cirrhosis. Clinical case. Rev Med Chil 2002;130(4):433–6.
36. Georgiou C, Neofytou K, Demetriades D. Local and systemic hemostatics as an adjunct to control bleeding in trauma. Am Surg 2013;79(2):180–7.

Retroperitoneal and Rectus Sheath Hematomas

George Kasotakis, MD, MPH

KEYWORDS

- Retroperitoneal • Rectus sheath • Hematomas • Retroperitoneum

KEY POINTS

- The retroperitoneum is rich in vascular structures and can harbor large hematomas, traumatic or spontaneous.
- The management of retroperitoneal hematomas depends on mechanism of injury and whether they are pulsatile/expanding.
- Rectus sheath hematomas are uncommon abdominal wall hematomas usually secondary to trauma to the epigastric arteries of the rectus muscle.
- Common risk factors include anticoagulation, strenuous exercise, coughing, coagulation disorders, and invasive procedures on/through the abdominal wall.
- The management is largely supportive, with reversal of anticoagulation and transfusions; angioembolization may be necessary.

RETROPERITONEAL HEMATOMAS

The retroperitoneum is an organ-rich region with several vital structures. It can be a site of major bleeding and harbor sizable hematomas caused by its highly vascular nature after trauma, surgical or endovascular interventions in the area, or spontaneously in patients on anticoagulation therapy or with vascular lesions.[1–4]

The retroperitoneum is divided in 3 anatomically distinct zones (**Fig. 1**): *Zone I*, or central retroperitoneal (RP), is defined as the area medial to the renal hila and contains the abdominal aorta and inferior vena cava, the celiac axis, superior mesenteric artery, and proximal renal vasculature. It also contains the pancreas and RP portion of the duodenum. *Zone II*, or lateral RP, includes the adrenals, the kidneys, and proximal genitourinary tract. *Zone III*, or pelvic RP, contains the rectum, the iliac vessels, and their branches/tributaries.[5]

Although in patients with multiple injuries a significant RP hemorrhage can manifest with hemodynamic instability and less commonly with ecchymoses in the affected areas, its clinical presentation in postprocedural or anticoagulated patients can be protean and include signs and symptoms such as malaise, unexplained tachycardia,

Section of Trauma & Acute Care Surgery, Boston Medical Center, Boston University School of Medicine, 840 Harrison Avenue, Dowling 2 South, #2414, Boston, MA 02118, USA
E-mail address: gkasot@bu.edu

Surg Clin N Am 94 (2014) 71–76
http://dx.doi.org/10.1016/j.suc.2013.10.007
0039-6109/14/$ – see front matter © 2014 Elsevier Inc. All rights reserved.

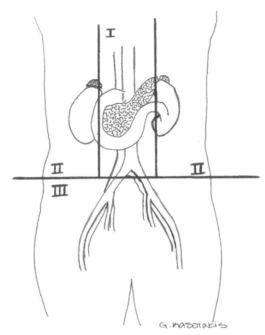

Fig. 1. The zones of the retroperitoneum.

a slowly dwindling hematocrit, hematuria, flank or back pain, ecchymoses, or even hypotension and abdominal compartment syndrome.

Although the diagnosis can easily be established with computed tomography, ideally with intravenous contrast that may detect active extravasation, the acute care surgeon should consider RP bleeding in hypotensive injured patients with normal chest and pelvic radiographs and a negative FAST (focused abdominal sonography for trauma).[2]

The management of RP hematomas, in addition to resuscitation and transfusions as needed, almost always revolves around surgical exploration in cases of spontaneous or postprocedural hemorrhage, with reversal of anticoagulation and angioembolization being useful adjuncts. Traumatic RP hematomas identified at laparotomy are explored depending on the mechanism of injury (blunt vs penetrating) and whether they are pulsatile or expanding.[6,7] All zone I RP hematomas mandate exploration, ideally after proximal (and when applicable, distal) control is established, to ensure no major vascular injuries are missed. Similarly, all RP hematomas after penetrating injuries should be explored, especially when major vessels are within the bullet/sharp object trajectory. Zone II and III RP bleeds after blunt injury should be explored only if pulsatile or expanding.[8] Should patients with hypotensive blunt trauma with severe pelvic fractures and a zone III hematoma require laparotomy, preperitoneal packing (usually with 3 laparotomy pads on either side of the bladder) can be undertaken through a separate low transverse incision, until angiography and embolization can be performed.[5,9,10]

Table 1 summarizes the management principles of RP hematomas.

RECTUS SHEATH HEMATOMAS

Rectus sheath hematoma (RSH) is a relatively uncommon condition, which arises from bleeding into the sheath of the rectus muscle, typically from trauma to the epigastric

Table 1
Management of RP hematomas identified at laparotomy

	Zone I (Central RP)	Zone II (Lateral RP)	Zone III (Pelvic RP)
Penetrating	Exploration	Exploration	Exploration/angiography
Blunt	Exploration	Exploration if expanding	Angiography/exploration if expanding

arteries or less commonly of the rectus muscle itself.[11,12] Most commonly it is localized below the arcuate line, where the posterior rectus sheath is absent and the epigastric vessels are relatively fixed and vulnerable to shearing forces.[13]

Although injury to the anterior abdominal wall is the most common triggering factor for RSH, spontaneous RSH is being encountered with increasing frequency.[12] Anticoagulation is the risk factor most commonly associated with spontaneous RSH, although other factors, such as antiplatelet therapy, advanced age, pregnancy, hypertension, recent abdominal surgery, and coagulation disorders, have also been described.[14–22]

Acute paroxysmal coughing seems to be the most common triggering factor, usually in patients with any of the aforementioned predisposing factors.[11] In addition to coughing, any condition that leads to a transient, sudden increase in intra-abdominal pressure, such as vomiting, straining during defecation or labor, and strenuous abdominal exercises, can cause RSH.[11,22] Women seem to be twice as prone to developing RSH as men because of the differences in muscle mass and stretching of their anterior abdominal wall associated with pregnancy.[23] RSH can also be iatrogenic after abdominal wall injections, paracenteses, or other invasive procedures through the lower anterior abdominal wall (**Fig. 2**).[24,25]

RSH typically presents with abdominal pain, usually progressively worsening as the hematoma enlarges, and a mass that does not cross the midline. Abdominal wall

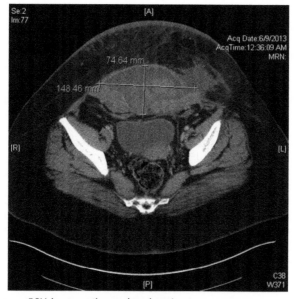

Fig. 2. Spontaneous RSH in an anticoagulated patient.

ecchymoses can often be appreciated on clinical examination.[11,26] Signs of acute blood loss (tachycardia, dizziness, orthostasis) are frequently present. The pain associated with RSH can worsen while lifting the shoulders from a supine position (Carnett sign), suggestive of abdominal wall pathology.[22] Smaller hematomas can become more evident on physical examination if patients contract the abdominal wall musculature by elevating their lower extremities while supine (Fothergill sign).[12] One or more of the previously discussed risk factors can usually be elicited in the history. Less commonly, a large RSH can present with hypotension, anemia, and even abdominal compartment syndrome.[27,28]

Diagnosis is established through consistent history and clinical examination findings and can be confirmed with ultrasonography or computed tomography. The latter can demonstrate active extravasation from the bleeding vessel if intravenous contrast is administered.

Even though most RSH are self-limiting with observation alone, they may lead to hemorrhagic shock in up to 37.5% of cases; mortality can be as high as 25%, particularly if associated with anticoagulation therapy.[12] In such severe cases, repeated transfusions and/or angioembolization of the bleeding vessel may be required.[29] Imaging-guided drainage can be considered in carefully selected cases; however, the risk of superinfection of the residual hematoma and rebleeding caused by the loss of the tamponade effect must be taken into consideration. Surgical evacuation is rarely appropriate because it may release the tamponade effect and is associated with significant morbidity.[22] It should be considered in cases when conservative management has failed and hemorrhage is ongoing or in the presence of compartment syndrome.[30]

REFERENCES

1. Sunga KL, Bellolio MF, Gilmore RM, et al. Spontaneous retroperitoneal hematoma: etiology, characteristics, management, and outcome. J Emerg Med 2012;43(2):e157–61.
2. Ernits M, Mohan PS, Fares LG 2nd, et al. A retroperitoneal bleed induced by enoxaparin therapy. Am Surg 2005;71(5):430–3.
3. Besir FH, Gul M, Ornek T, et al. Enoxaparin-associated giant retroperitoneal hematoma in pulmonary embolism treatment. N Am J Med Sci 2011;3(11):524–6.
4. Kim YH, Kim CK, Park CB, et al. Spontaneous rupture of internal iliac artery secondary to anticoagulant therapy. Ann Thorac Cardiovasc Surg 2013;19(3): 228–30.
5. Britt LD, Maxwell RA. Chapter 12. Management of abdominal trauma. In: Zinner MJ, Ashley SW, editors. Maingot's abdominal operations. 12th edition. New York: McGraw-Hill; 2013. Available at: http://www.accesssurgery.com. ezproxy.bu.edu/content.aspx?aID=57008151. Accessed July 8, 2013.
6. Chan YC, Morales JP, Reidy JF, et al. Management of spontaneous and iatrogenic retroperitoneal haemorrhage: conservative management, endovascular intervention or open surgery? Int J Clin Pract 2008;62(10):1604–13.
7. Ali J. Chapter 95. Torso trauma. In: Hall JB, Schmidt GA, Wood LD, editors. Principles of critical care. 3rd edition. New York: McGraw-Hill; 2005. Available at: http://www.accesssurgery.com.ezproxy.bu.edu/content.aspx?aID=2298290. Accessed July 8, 2013.
8. Feliciano DV. Management of traumatic retroperitoneal hematoma. Ann Surg 1990;211(2):109–23.
9. Burlew CC, Moore EE, Smith WR, et al. Preperitoneal pelvic packing/external fixation with secondary angioembolization: optimal care for life-threatening

hemorrhage from unstable pelvic fractures. J Am Coll Surg 2011;212(4):628–35 [discussion: 635–7].

10. Cothren CC, Moore EE, Smith WR, et al. Preperitoneal pelvic packing in the child with an unstable pelvis: a novel approach. J Pediatr Surg 2006;41(4): e17–9.

11. Cherry WB, Mueller PS. Rectus sheath hematoma: review of 126 cases at a single institution. Medicine 2006;85(2):105–10.

12. Smithson A, Ruiz J, Perello R, et al. Diagnostic and management of spontaneous rectus sheath hematoma. Eur J Intern Med 2013;24(6):579–82.

13. Edlow JA, Burstein J. Rectus sheath hematoma. Ann Emerg Med 2000;36(1):79.

14. Gabel A, Muller S. Fatal hematoma during treatment with adjusted-dose subcutaneous heparin therapy. N Engl J Med 1999;340(1):61–2.

15. Lambroza A, Tighe MK, DeCosse JJ, et al. Disorders of the rectus abdominis muscle and sheath: a 22-year experience. Am J Gastroenterol 1995;90(8): 1313–7.

16. Girolami A, Allemand E, Tezza F, et al. Rectus muscle sheath haematoma in a patient with congenital FX deficiency and in another with congenital FVII deficiency. Haemophilia 2010;16(1):182–5.

17. Fitzgerald JE, Fitzgerald LA, Anderson FE, et al. The changing nature of rectus sheath haematoma: case series and literature review. Int J Surg 2009;7(2): 150–4.

18. Fujikawa T, Kawato M, Tanaka A. Spontaneous rectus sheath haematoma caused by warfarin-induced overanticoagulation. BMJ Case Rep 2011;2011. pii: bcr0720114533.

19. Tolcher MC, Nitsche JF, Arendt KW, et al. Spontaneous rectus sheath hematoma pregnancy: case report and review of the literature. Obstet Gynecol Surv 2010; 65(8):517–22.

20. Salemis NS. Spontaneous rectus sheath hematoma presenting as acute surgical abdomen: an important differential in elderly coagulopathic patients. Geriatr Gerontol Int 2009;9(2):200–2.

21. Denard PJ, Fetter JC, Zacharski LR. Rectus sheath hematoma complicating low-molecular weight heparin therapy. Int J Lab Hematol 2007;29(3):190–4.

22. Donaldson J, Knowles CH, Clark SK, et al. Rectus sheath haematoma associated with low molecular weight heparin: a case series. Ann R Coll Surg Engl 2007; 89(3):309–12.

23. Dubinsky IL. Hematoma of the rectus abdominis muscle: case report and review of the literature. J Emerg Med 1997;15(2):165–7.

24. Parkinson F, Khalid U, Woolgar J. Rectus sheath haematoma: a serious complication of a commonly administered drug. BMJ Case Rep 2013;2013. pii: bcr2012008183.

25. Laohapensang K, Sirivanichai C. An unusual complication of EVAR, spontaneous rectus sheath hematoma: a case report. Ann Vasc Dis 2009;2(2):122–5.

26. Sahin M, Coskun S, Cobanoglu M, et al. Rapidly onset rectus sheath hematoma mimicking cholecystitis. Am J Emerg Med 2011;29(6):698.e5–8.

27. Shokoohi H, Boniface K, Reza Taheri M, et al. Spontaneous rectus sheath hematoma diagnosed by point-of-care ultrasonography. CJEM 2013;15(2): 119–22.

28. McBeth PB, Dunham M, Ball CG, et al. Correct the coagulopathy and scoop it out: complete reversal of anuric renal failure through the operative decompression of extraperitoneal hematoma-induced abdominal compartment syndrome. Case Rep Med 2012;2012:946103.

29. Rimola J, Perendreu J, Falco J, et al. Percutaneous arterial embolization in the management of rectus sheath hematoma. AJR Am J Roentgenol 2007;188(6): W497–502.
30. Jafferbhoy SF, Rustum Q, Shiwani MH. Abdominal compartment syndrome–a fatal complication from a rectus sheath haematoma. BMJ Case Rep 2012;2012. pii:bcr1220115332.

Acute Obstruction

Jason Sperry, MD, MPH[a], Mitchell Jay Cohen, MD[b],*

KEYWORDS

- Acute care surgery • Acute obstruction • Adhesions • Ischemia • Volvulus
- Cholangitis

KEY POINTS

- Acute gastric outlet obstruction secondary to paraesophageal hernia or gastric volvulus is a surgical emergency.
- Laparoscopic manage of small bowel obstruction secondary to adhesions has been demonstrated to be safe and potentially lower morbidity and length of stay.
- Patients with small bowel obstruction without risks of adhesions require a low threshold for early operative intervention.
- Treatment of colonic obstruction is dependent on degree (complete vs partial), anatomic location, and etiology.
- Biliary obstruction with infection (cholangitis) requires emergent drainage and is primarily treated via nonsurgical (ERCP or PTC) means.

OBSTRUCTION

Acute obstruction of the gastrointestinal or biliary tract represents a common problem for acute care surgeons and necessitates focused attention to patients' presentation, physical examination, laboratory and radiographic evaluation, and prior history. The spectrum of management options for these difficult pathologic processes ranges from conservative decompression through expeditious operative intervention depending on the anatomic location of obstruction, the nature and rapidity of symptom presentation, and the prior surgical history of patients. It is with appropriate clinical evaluation, planning, and physical examination follow-up that acute care surgeons are able to appropriately diagnose, manage, and resolve this difficult group of surgical problems and minimize the morbidity associated with each.

Presentation of Acute Esophageal Obstruction

Acute esophageal obstruction most commonly arises from foreign body impaction, either in association with a preexisting esophageal disorder or process, accidental

[a] University of Pittsburgh Medical Center, Suite F1268 PUH, 200 Lothrop Street, Pittsburgh, PA 15213, USA; [b] Department of Surgery, San Francisco General Hospital, University of California San Francisco, 1001 Potrero Avenue, San Francisco, CA 94110, USA
* Corresponding author.
E-mail address: mcohen@sfghsurg.ucsf.edu

Surg Clin N Am 94 (2014) 77–96
http://dx.doi.org/10.1016/j.suc.2013.10.001
0039-6109/14/$ – see front matter © 2014 Elsevier Inc. All rights reserved.
surgical.theclinics.com

ingestion, or in some cases intentional ingestion.[1] Acute foreign body impaction is a gastrointestinal emergency and can be associated with significant morbidity and even mortality due to complications, including aspiration and esophageal injury or perforation.[2] The most common cause of foreign body obstruction in adults is meat bolus impaction above a preexisting esophageal condition. Underlying esophageal conditions commonly include esophageal mucosal (Schatzki) rings, peptic or malignant strictures, eosinophilic esophagitis, or achalasia.[3,4] A majority of adults are symptomatic; symptoms can occur within minutes to hours after ingestion. Acute dysphagia and inability to tolerate saliva are key symptoms in addition to retrosternal fullness, hiccups, or retching. Inability to swallow saliva typically indicates complete esophageal obstruction and requires urgent attention whereas odynophagia should elicit concerns for esophageal laceration or perforation.[5] Respiratory symptoms, including stridor, dyspnea, or cough, can result from tracheal compression, particularly in younger patients, whereas aspiration risk is elevated in those with complete esophageal obstruction.

Diagnosis and evaluation

Clinical examination on presentation provides the primary impetus for further evaluation. Radiologic evaluation helps confirm clinical suspicion and can confirm location and associated complications. Plain films of the neck, chest, and abdominal radiogrpahs are typically needed and may demonstrate a radiopaque foreign body. Findings of mediastinal, subdiaphramatic, subcutaneous air, or pleural effusion all suggest complications associated with acute esophageal obstruction, including perforation.[6] Importantly, meat impaction or other nonradiopaque foreign bodies are not visualized on plain film, and failure to localize on plain film does not preclude its presence. In those patients with a stable or controlled airway, CT imaging is superior to plain radiographs for foreign body detection, characterization (size, shape, and perforation concern), and management decision options. Contrast swallow evaluation should not be performed due to the increased risk of aspiration.

Management

Simultaneously with history and physical, airway protection and management are of the utmost importance.[7] Those patients with respiratory symptoms and inability to tolerate secretions should be endotracheally intubated. Medical management, including glucagon administration, has been described for food bolus impaction; however, the literature remains conflicted regarding its actual benefit and caution should be used in those patients with underlying esophageal pathology, such as strictures or malignancy, resulting in an underlying fixed obstruction.[2,8] The mainstay of treatment of acute esophageal obstruction is endoscopy evaluation and retrieval.[9] Flexible endoscopy under conscious sedation or general anesthesia is the procedure of choice, with success rates of more than 90% in the recent literature. Rigid esophagoscopy requires general anesthesia and is preferable in younger patients and in those patients with sharp object impaction or obstruction. Blunt objects that have passed into the stomach can usually be managed conservatively. Gentle pushing of a food bolus into the stomach can be attempted. Simultaneous evaluation for strictures or esophageal pathology should be undertaken. Sharp objects require urgent attention to reduce the risk of perforation. Special attention to impacted disc or button batteries due to the risk of caustic injury and perforation is required.[1,2,9]

Once the acute obstruction has been appropriately evaluated and definitively managed, an underlying esophageal process that led to the obstruction should be sought. This may require additional endoscopic examination, thoracic CT imaging, esophageal manometry, or flouroscopic esophageal contrast evaluation.

Similar evaluation for those esophageal processes, which present with a more indolent presentation or subacute obstruction, should be performed.

Presentation of Acute Gastric Outlet Obstruction

Presentation
Patients with acute gastric obstruction present most commonly with a variable combination of symptoms, including epigastric pain, nausea, and vomiting. The prior medical and surgical history of patients is extremely important for this relatively nonspecific surgical presentation. Prior history of peptic ulcer disease, pancreatitis, or hiatal hernia; prior surgical history; and the time course for the presenting symptoms provide essential information to acute care surgeons, allowing appropriate management of this difficult problem. Those patients who present with peritonitis and signs and symptoms of shock or sepsis require urgent surgical evaluation with a concern for possible bowel strangulation or perforation.[10,11]

Diagnosis and evaluation
An acute abdominal series, which includes a flat and upright abdominal plain film radiographs, is commonly obtained in patients who present with abdominal pain, nausea, or vomiting. Bowel dilatation can efficiently be assessed as well as free intra-abdominal air or gastric dilatation or gastric air fluid level. These images can be obtained early while initiation of resuscitation and possible nasogastric decompression, in those patients with vomiting or signs of dehydration, is begun.[12-15] Causes of acute gastric outlet or proximal duodenal obstruction can be categorized into extrinsic compression, intrinsic obstruction, intraluminal obstruction, or secondary to acute incarceration or strangulation. Extrinsic compression and gastric or proximal duodenal obstruction can result from pancreatitis, associated pseudocyst formation, or hematoma compression.[10] Intrinsic causes include malignancy and peptic ulcer disease and associated strictures. Intraluminal obstruction can result from gastric bezoars, intentional ingestion of foreign bodies, gallstones, or, similar to acute esophageal obstruction, food impaction with an underlying gastric or proximal duodenal pathologic process.[16-18] The acute incarceration or strangulation category consists of acute paraesophageal hernias presenting with obstruction or acute gastric volvulus.[11,19] The management options and requirements for each category of acute gastric obstruction vary, with the acute incarceration or strangulation category requiring the most expeditious acute surgical evaluation and intervention. In those patients without an acute abdomen, peritonitis, or urgent requirement for the operating room, abdominal CT imaging should be performed and is the gold standard for evaluating epigastric pain, nausea, vomiting, and the cause of acute gastric obstruction. The addition of an upper gastrointestinal contrast study may assist in the characterization of acute gastric outlet obstruction when the diagnosis remains poorly characterized.[20] Additionally, laboratory evaluation can provide insight into the severity and time course of an upper gastrointestinal obstruction based on the severity of metabolic acid/base abnormalities.

Management
Management should include aggressive resuscitation based on the presenting history and status of a patient. Radiographic evaluation allows characterization of the etiology of the acute gastric outlet obstruction. External compression and intrinsic gastric obstruction mechanisms typically can be managed with nasogastric decompression and initial conservative management while further work-up and evaluation of the extrinsic or intrinsic pathology is performed. These should include upper gastrointestinal contrast examination and endoscopy. Patients with pancreatitis and or

pseudocyst-induced gastric obstruction should be placed on short-term bowel rest; endoscopic feeding access can be placed using a nasogastric jejunal double lumen tube, which allows gastric decompression and distal feeding access; and formal evaluation of the pancreatic duct and other pancreatitis complications should be undertaken when indicated.[10] Patients with gastric strictures resulting from peptic ulcer disease or malignancy resulting in acute gastric obstruction require nasogastric decompression, gastric acid suppression, endoscopic evaluation, biopsy, and definitive preoperative surgical evaluation. Endoscopic balloon dilatation also is increasingly used for obstruction secondary to peptic ulcer disease.[21] Endoscopic expandable wall stents may increasingly play a role most commonly in patients with advanced malignancy when palliative relief of obstruction is required.[22,23] Operative management may include definitive gastric resection or gastrojejunostomy based on the underlying pathologic process. Again, enteral distal feeding access, if able to be obtained, has been shown beneficial for those patients who require definitive operative intervention or in those in whom conservative managed is undertaken.

Intraluminal gastric outlet obstruction is primarily evaluated and managed via endoscopic techniques. Bezoars may require endoscopic fragmentation, whereas sharp foreign bodies or batteries should be removed endoscopically.[18] Those foreign bodies that require removal but are unable to be endoscopically removed require operative removal with a gastrotomy via an epigastric approach.

Patients who present with acute gastric outlet obstruction secondary to either paraesophageal hernia or gastric volvulus are surgical emergencies and should be evaluated expeditiously. Historically, an open operative approach has been the standard but, increasingly, series of laprascopic managed acute paraesophageal incarcerations and gastric volvulus have demonstrated the safety and feasible of this practice. In those cases where perforation or necrosis of the stomach is found, conversion to open is recommended. For the operative approach for paraesophageal hernia, standard tenets of operative management should be followed, including reduction of the hernia, resection of sac, crural closure, and fundoplication. Clinical status, age of the patients, and hemodynamic stability typically determine the full extent of either the laparoscopic or open repair. A gastropexy for those patients with gastric volvulus is commonly required and can also be performed laparoscopically in a well-described safe fashion.

ADHESIONAL AND NONADHESIONAL SMALL BOWEL OBSTRUCTION

Small bowel obstruction represents an exceedingly common and persistent problem for acute care surgeons manage and accounts for up to 15% of all surgical admissions to US hospitals. Similar to other gastrointestinal obstructions, the presentation, physical examination, radiographic and laboratory evaluation, and surgical history represent essential information to appropriately manage this surgical process.[24,25] The risk of bowel strangulation and ischemia represents the primary driver for early operative intervention. Prior operative exposure or risk of peritoneal adhesions represents the first major branch point in the decision process algorithm for the management of small bowel obstruction because these two different cohorts of patients should be evaluated and managed differently, specifically for the expeditious need for operative intervention.[26–28]

Presentation of Adhesional Small Bowel Obstruction

Small bowel obstruction in patients with prior abdominal procedures with a risk of abdominal adhesions commonly present with a variable combination of symptoms, including abdominal pain and distension, nausea, and vomiting. The rapidity at which symptoms present and order in which symptoms arise is important to elicit as are the specific abdominal surgery history and timing of those prior procedures.[26,29] A history of prior hernias or recent abdominal or groin mass is essential information because a small bowel obstruction resulting from a hernia is high on the differential and needs to be investigated. Those patients who present with peritonitis and signs and symptoms of shock or sepsis require urgent surgical evaluation with a concern for possible bowel strangulation or perforation resulting from a closed loop small bowel obstruction.[27]

Diagnosis and evaluation

Acute abdominal series, which includes flat and upright abdominal plain film radiographs, are commonly obtained in patients who present with small bowel obstruction symptoms, abdominal distension, or pain. Small bowel and colonic dilatation can be assessed efficiently as well as free intra-abdominal air via an acute abdominal series. These can be obtained early while initiation of resuscitation and possible nasogastric decompression, in those patients with vomiting or signs of dehydration, is begun.[12–15] Based on physical examination, history, and further laboratory evaluation, abdominal CT imaging should be obtained in those patients without need for more urgent operative intervention and in whom an obstructive process is a concern.[26,27,30]

Abdominal CT has increasingly become the gold standard for evaluation of small bowel obstruction due to its higher sensitivity and risk stratification abilities compared with other modalities.[31,32] Oral and intravenous contrast provides improved bowel and viscera evaluation in those patients without contrast contraindications; however, cautious use of oral contrast should be used in those patients with significant vomiting or distension and who have an associated high risk of aspiration. The utility of abdominal CT imaging comes from its ability to provide information regarding bowel strangulation or ischemia and characterize small bowel transition areas into partial or low-grade obstructions and complete or high-grade obstructions.[33] This radiographic differentiation is important because complete or high-grade small bowel obstructions are associated with up a 20% to 40% incidence of bowel strangulation.[26,27] Abdominal CT findings, which should raise suspicion of small bowel ischemia, include intra-abdominal free fluid, small bowel fecalization, mesenteric edema, lack of small bowel mucosal enhancement when intravenous contrast is used, and swirling mesentery, suggesting small bowel volvulus (**Fig. 1**).[34–36]

In addition to physical examination and radiographic assessment, laboratory evaluation can provide important information regarding the risk of small bowel strangulation and ischemia and can help decipher the need for urgent operative intervention. Historically, leukocytosis, metabolic acidosis, and elevated serum lactate levels are well-described risk factors of bowel ischemia, although they lack specificity and can be elevated for a broad range of pathologic processes.[37–39] More recent evidence suggests that measurements of serum procalcitonin may predict bowel ischemia and those patients who may fail conservative management of small bowel obstruction.[40] There remains a significant need for serum biomarkers, which have both a high sensitivity and specificity for bowel ischemia. Currently, however, laboratory evaluation remains nonspecific but provides additional information that can aid acute care surgeons in determining the best management option when evaluating patients with acute small bowel obstruction.

Management

Management decisions should be based on clinical presentation and physical examination, radiographic imaging, and laboratory evaluation (**Fig. 2**).[41,42] The risk for bowel

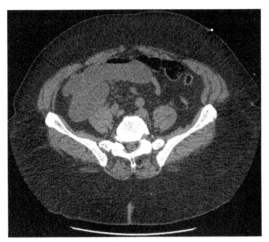

Fig. 1. High-grade small bowel obstruction from adhesions.

strangulation and ischemia represents the principle factor dictating the early decision process.[43] Management options include surgical management, including both laparoscopic and open operative approaches, and conservative management with nasogastric decompression and serial examinations.[28,44] An increasing pool of literature suggests that a laparoscopic approach for management of adhesive small bowel obstruction is feasible and effective and can be accomplished with acceptable

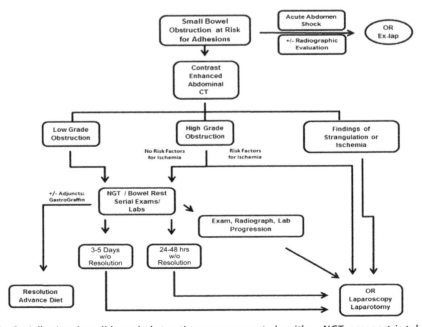

Fig. 2. Adhesional small bowel obstruction management algorithm. NGT, nasogastric tube.

morbidity.[44–47] In one of the largest reviews on this topic, an initial laparoscopic approach was successful in 64% of cases with another 6% managed as laparoscopy assisted. The remaining 30% were converted to midline laparotomy for reasons including dense adhesions, bowel resection, unidentified pathology, and iatrogenic injury.[48] The laparoscopic approach has been touted primarily for its associated lower morbidity and shorter length of stay.[49,50]

Those patients with CT findings concerning for strangulation or ischemia or high grade with risk factors for ischemia should undergo operative intervention via a laparoscopic or laparotomy approach, depending on the patient anatomy and prior surgical history. In those stable patients with low-grade or high-grade obstruction with no other risk factors for bowel ischemia or strangulation, a conservative management approach with gastric decompression and bowel risk is safe and appropriate.[24,26,27] In those patients who undergo attempted conservative management, close serial evaluation is essential. Serial physical examinations, laboratory evaluation, and even repeat radiographic imaging can be used to determine whether resolution of the small bowel obstruction is occurring or whether conservative management has failed. High-level evidence suggests that oral Gastrografin and follow-up imaging, in those patients who have not significantly improved from an obstruction standpoint in the first 48 hours, may provide both diagnostic and therapeutic benefit by determining those patients likely to fail conservative management, a reduction in the need for surgery, and shorter length of stay.[51–54] Surgical intervention should occur in those with worsening physical examination or laboratory markers or who undergo radiographic imaging suggesting persistent or new findings concerning for bowel ischemia or strangulation. Due to the greater risk of bowel strangulation and ischemia with high-grade obstructions, up to 40% is most series, a low threshold for operative intervention over the first 24 to 48 hours is required if the obstruction does not resolve or symptoms progress.[42,43,55,56] The timing at which operative intervention should occur for those stable patients with low-grade obstruction who fail to improve remains controversial, with a majority of literature and recent evidenced-based guidelines suggesting that waiting beyond 3 to 5 days is associated with worse overall outcome.[55,57] Evidence regarding the management of early postoperative obstruction (<30 days from prior laparotomy) suggests that the majority can be managed expectantly. Some investigators support that beyond 6 to 14 days of failed conservative management operative intervention is likely beneficial.[58–61] On the other hand, an operation at this period may become extremely challenging, because inflammatory adhesion formation is at its peak and injury to important structures may occur. It requires a careful balance of advantages and disadvantages to make the decision for an operation and, no matter the decision, it potentially is the wrong one (**Fig. 3**).

Presentation of Nonadhesional Small Bowel Obstruction

In those patients without a prior history of abdominal operation or risk factors for adhesions, small bowel obstruction presents in a similar fashion to those with adhesional obstruction, including a variable combination of symptoms, including abdominal pain and distension, nausea, and vomiting. Because adhesions are not the likely cause of the obstructive symptoms, a thorough hernia examination should be performed to rule out bowel incarceration as the cause of the obstruction. Again, those patients with peritonitis or signs and symptoms of shock should undergo urgent surgical evaluation with a concern for possible bowel strangulation or perforation (**Fig. 4**).[26,29]

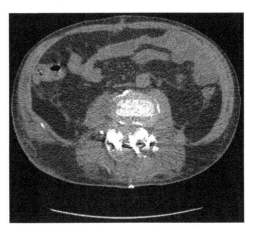

Fig. 3. Low-grade small bowel obstruction from adhesions.

Diagnosis and evaluation

Without adhesions as the cause of obstruction, age-specific alternative small bowel obstructing causes in addition to hernia should be considered, including internal hernia, malignancy, gallstone ileus, bezoar, Meckel diverticulum, inflammatory bowel disease, stricture, malrotation, and volvulus. Irrespective of the cause of the obstruction

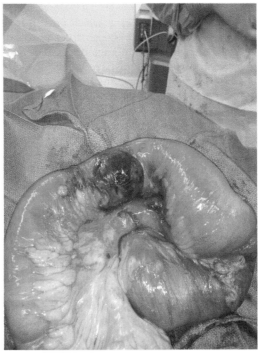

Fig. 4. High-grade small bowel obstruction without adhesion risk factors due to spontaneous hematoma.

and similar to adhesional small bowel obstruction, radiographic abdominal evaluation with initial plain films and enhanced CT imaging provides important characterization of the small bowel obstruction, which has direct management implications. Laboratory evaluation similarly provides additional information regarding the risk of bowel strangulation or ischemia and should be followed serially in those who are managed initially via a conservative approach.

Management

As with small bowel obstruction due to adhesions, management decisions should be based on clinical presentation and physical examination, radiographic imaging, and laboratory evaluation (**Fig. 5**), with the risk for bowel strangulation and ischemia representing the principle factor dictating the early decision process.[26,27,62] Although adhesional obstruction has a high rate of successful conservative management, patients without risks of adhesions require a low threshold for operative intervention.[24] Patients who present with peritonitis and signs and symptoms of shock or sepsis require expeditious operative intervention typically via a laparotomy approach. Patients who can be afforded further characterization of the obstruction with contrast-enhanced CT imaging can be stratified into those with low-grade or partial obstruction, with high-grade or complete obstruction, and with concerning findings of bowel strangulation or ischemia.[26,27] Patients with CT findings of bowel strangulation or ischemia require expeditious surgical intervention.[56] Even those stable patients

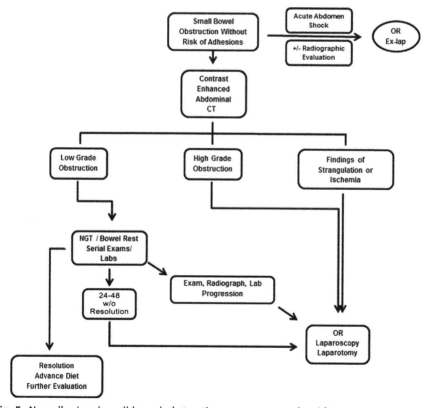

Fig. 5. Nonadhesional small bowel obstruction management algorithm.

with high-grade obstruction on CT imaging should undergo early surgical intervention due to the high likelihood of bowel strangulation, ischemia, or requirement for resection when adhesions are not the cause for the obstruction. Patients who remain stable with low-grade or partial obstructions and no other concerning laboratory risk factors for ischemia can undergo a short trial of conservative management with a low threshold to convert to operative management over the first 24 to 48 hours if progression of examination, radiographs, or laboratory results worsen or if patients fail to resolve the obstruction.[33,34,62] Further radiographic or endoscopic evaluation for inflammatory bowel disease or malignancy during this short window of nonoperative management may assist in planning subsequent interventions. In those patients who resolve, an aggressive evaluation for the cause of the nonadhesional obstruction is required, which may include diagnostic laparoscopy irrespective of obstructive symptom resolution.[26,27]

Presentation of Acute Colonic Obstruction

Acute colonic obstruction is a surgical emergency, which requires the skills of an acute care surgeon to make rapid diagnosis and effect quick management to resuscitate the patient and relieve the obstruction. As with small bowel obstruction, the presentation is one of increasing abdominal distention, nausea, vomiting, malaise, reduced flatus and stool, and eventually obstipation. Depending on the acuity of the obstruction and the anatomic location, the constellation of symptoms can vary and any of these symptoms may be prevalent or absent. Because the early symptomatology can mimic or be mimicked by many other disease processes, a high index and broad differential index of suspicion are necessary to diagnose. Causes and, hence, presentations of large bowel obstruction can be divided into mechanical or functional. Mechanical causes can be further subdivided into anatomic (torsion or volvulus or fecal impaction) benign inflammatory (diverticulitis/pancreatitis), or malignancy.[63] The onset of symptoms from mechanical obstruction can range from sudden without any precedent (torsion or volvulus) to slow and indolent (fecal impaction). Sigmoid and cecal volvulus often has a specific time of initiation, which can be delineated with a careful history.[64] Inflammatory and malignant causes of colonic obstruction often have disease-specific symptoms, which precede the actual colonic obstruction, which also can be delineated by a careful history and physical examination.

Diagnosis

Diagnosis begins with a complete history and physical examination. Although unfortunately becoming a lost art, the cause and level of the colonic obstruction can be often discerned by an astute diagnostician with a careful history and physical examination. Mechanical anatomic causes (volvulus and torsion) often have a specific beginning of symptoms, which can be delineated on history.[64] Although patients often initially describe an indolent course with careful questioning, they often reveal a specific beginning of symptoms. In contrast, inflammatory and malignant causes have a diversity of symptomatology that can range from slow and indolent with episodes of partial obstruction or abdominal pain, which spontaneously resolve for days to months prior to presentation with complete obstruction. At the most extreme range, patients present with perforation and peritonitis. Patients with an obvious surgical abdomen need little or no further diagnosis and should be resuscitated and proceed directly to the operating room.

After history and physical examination, imaging studies are warranted. Radiologic imaging most often should begin with plain abdominal films. Usually referred to as an obstructive series or 3 views of the abdomen, these consist of a complete interrogation of the abdomen both upright and supine. Plain films can often determine the degree of abdominal distention and location of distention (without specificity) and evaluate for free perforation. In particular, sigmoid volvulus can be diagnosed 50% to 70% of the time on plain radiographs with a characteristic finding of a bent inner tube appearance.[64] Despite common belief of the existence of a radiologic signature, cecal volvulus plain radiographs can facilitate the diagnosis in only one-quarter of patients and the diagnosis is usually made on CT scan.[65,66]

Although an important first step, plain films most often cannot often determine cause of obstruction, and additional imaging in stable patients is needed and warranted. That said, evidence of cecal or colonic diameter of greater than 13 cm, extraluminal free air, or the radiologic diagnosis of large bowel volvulus is a cause to proceed directly to treatment.

When plain films are not directly diagnostic and there is no cause to proceed directly to exploration, additional imaging is warranted. A contrast study from above or below was for many years the gold standard for diagnosis. An upper gastrointestinal contrast study with small bowel follow through was most often used to determine the level and degree of obstruction. This test, used less often, is still warranted, especially when there is a question of completeness or level of obstruction. These studies, although dynamic and providing information on the degree and anatomic location of obstruction, are often not able to determine the cause of obstruction and cannot evaluate the extent of inflammatory or malignant pathology, which surrounds the bowel. As a result, these studies have largely been replaced by CT scan. Appropriately done, a CT scan can[65,66] identify both the level and cause of obstruction.

Along with imaging, comprehensive laboratory tests should be sent to evaluate for other diagnostic markers (inflammatory) as well as electrolyte abnormalities to guide resuscitation.

Management
Like any broad topic, management depends on the underlying pathology and level of obstruction. Ultimately, however, some broad truths exist. Any patient with perforation or peritonitis needs acute resuscitation and surgical exploration. In these cases, the operative approach varies depending on the anatomic nature of the obstruction and the degree of physiologic derangement. In each case, these range from resection with primary anastomosis to damage control laparotomy (discussed later).

Patients with partial or subacute obstruction should be treated with nasogastric tube decompression and fluid resuscitation. A Foley catheter should be placed and laboratory results assessed (described previously) to determine the degree of resuscitation. The role of antibiotics is controversial. Any patient with diagnosed infectious or inflammatory causes of large bowel obstruction should be treated with broad-spectrum antibiotics, which are then narrowed as diagnosis and culture become more certain. The role of antibiotics in malignant, functional, or benign inflammatory obstruction remains unproved and they should only be given when suspicion for systemic disease or related infectious cause exists.

Although a complete treatise on the management of each cause of bowel obstruction is beyond the scope of this article, the following specific recommendations about treatment exist (**Fig. 6**).

Diverticulitis
Partial Treatment of diverticulitis complicated by obstruction centers on whether the obstruction is complete or partial and is further determined by the degree of colonic and extracolonic inflammation.[67] Fortunately, in most cases of diverticulitis, colonic

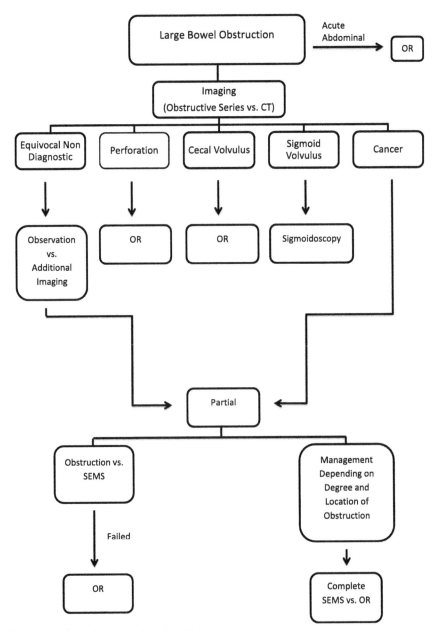

Fig. 6. Large bowel obstruction algorithm.

obstruction is partial. In cases of partial obstruction without peritonitis or perforation necessitating operative treatment, treatment of the underlying inflammation with bowel rest and antibiotics can often resolve the obstruction without surgery.[68] Decompression with nasogastric tube and fluid resuscitation along with broad-spectrum antibiotics (narrowed when specificities are available) is combined with careful observation. Failure to resolve the obstruction or progression of symptoms is then declared a failure of management and the treatment progresses to that of complete obstruction.

Complete In cases of complete obstruction (fortunately uncommon in diverticulitis) in physiologically stable patients, short periods of expectant management can be attempted. As with partial obstruction, the goal is treatment of underlying inflammation with the hope of converting a complete obstruction into a partial one allowing either no-operative treatment or preparation and elective delayed treatment.[69] This is accomplished (as described previously) with treatment of underlying inflammation, bowel rest, and antibiotics. If conversion to partial obstruction is successful, then treatment and observation are continued. If unsuccessful, then patients require laparotomy. At laparotomy, the degree of inflammation, local and distant, determines the operation done, which ranges from resection with primary anastomosis to resection with proximal diversion to proximal diversion without resection and distal drainage.[63,70]

Malignant Malignant disease of the colon is fraught with morbidity; 10% to 30% of colon cancers present with obstructing lesions, with a dismal associated 5-year survival rate of 20%.[71] Although the primary disease and/or oncologic severity certainty plays a role in poor outcomes, emergent surgery by itself is fraught with incumbent morbidity and worsened outcome. In reference to colon surgery, several groups have compared emergent surgery with elective surgery and noted mortality decreases from 20% to 25% with emergent surgery compared with 0.9% to 10% for elective surgery on similarly ill patients. As a result, temporization of the need for operation and the ability to convert an emergent situation into an urgent or semielective one is paramount. As with benign inflammatory causes, the degree of obstruction and physiologic obstruction determines the urgency and operative approach.

Partial In patients with who are physiologically stable, a partially obstructed malignancy can be observed with bowel rest, nasogastric tube decompression, and fluid resuscitation while staging and operative planning occur.[72] Specifics on the operative plan depend on the malignancy and are beyond the scope of this article.

Complete When there is a complete obstruction, surgical or stent-based relief of the obstruction is urgently indicated. Traditionally, this has necessitated laparotomy and proximal diversion with resection in cases of colon or proximal diversion without resection as a first stage toward neoadjuvant therapy in rectal cancer. When there is significant, pericolic inflammation, presence of perforation or abscess, or physiologic perturbation, conservative staged resection with proximal diversion is indicated.[72] In cases of complete obstruction without any mitigating issues and in stable patients with good physiology, resection with primary anastomosis can be completed. Although this has been the traditional approach and remains the standard of care, there recently has been new interest in the use of self-expanding stents (usually metallic) for the palliation or temporary relief of near-obstructing or obstructing colon lesions.[73,74] Several groups have reported on the use of self-expanding metal stents (SEMS) for the palliation of obstructing and near-obstructing colon masses. In the colon, placement is done by fluoroscopy, endoscopy, or a combined approach. Stents are introduced through the anus and guided either by the endoscope or via a wire and fluoroscopy. A combination of plain radiographs, CT, water-soluble contrast lower gastrointestinal imaging, and colonoscopy is used for preplacement planning. Generally a wire is placed across the obstructing lesion and the stent deployed. Fluoroscopy or less often endoscopy is used to confirm patency and the proximal and distal landing zones.

To date, there is a dearth of randomized controlled data on this subject, and most of the randomized trials are subject to considerable selection bias; however, many groups have reported the ability of stents to turn a functionally complete obstruction into a partial obstruction, allowing time for patient resuscitation and preparation and, thereby, turning an emergent situation into an urgent or elective one with resultant better outcomes.[73–76]

Inflammatory (pancreatitis) In colon obstruction secondary to pancreatitis, the treatment generally centers around treatment of the pancreatic inflammation. Rarely is it necessary to operate primarily on the colon.

Sigmoid volvulus Sigmoid volvulus is generally treated with sigmoidscopic decompression and untwisting of the torsed sigmoid colon. Because most sigmoid volvulus occurs in the distal 30 cm of colon, gentle insertion and insufflation with a sigmoid scope is sufficient to untwist and relieve the obstruction in 80% to 100% of cases.[77] Alternatively, a small percentage of these cases can be resolved with a contrast enema.[77] Some investigators have advocated the concurrent placement of a rectal tube to avoid rapid recurrence and facilitate additional decompression; however, this practice is not standard. Although sigmoidoscopy is generally rapidly successful, there remains a high recurrence rate; 40% to 60% of patients reoccur over days to months; hence, most investigators advocate urgent bowel preparation and sigmoid resection and sigmoidopexy.[64] In cases where initial decompression is unsuccessful or where perturbed physiology suggests necrosis or perforation, immediate laparotomy with resection and anastomosis or Hartmann procedure is indicated.

Cecal volvulus Cecal volvulus requires laparotomy, detorsion, and resection with either primary anastomosis or diversion (again depending on the state of the bowel).[65,66] In selected cases, cecopexy can be attempted with appendectomy (where adhesions fix the bowel), direct pexy, or cecostomy tube used to secure the colon.

Presentation of Acute Biliary Obstruction

Acute biliary obstruction occurs most often as a result of stone disease. Although it can also occur from malignancy, malignant disease most often presents indolently, resulting in painless partial then total obstruction and painless jaundice. Therefore, acute obstruction is most often the result of stone disease, which accounts for 50% to 70% of cases and likely a higher percentage in true acute obstruction. Other causes include malignancy, nonmalignant stricture, and rarely extrinsic compression. Acute obstruction is manifest by colicky abdominal pain, puritis nausea and vomiting, and, less often and later, by jaundice. In cases of cholangitis where the obstruction is complicated by infection, these symptoms are accompanied by fever, jaundice, and abdominal pain in 50% to 75% of patients.[78] The addition of mental status changes and hypotension to these symptoms constitutes Reynolds pentad and can often progress if untreated to organ failure and death.[65,66,79,80]

Diagnosis

Diagnosis is made beginning with a complete history and physical examination, which can often completely confer the diagnosis without additional testing. Laboratory tests, including biliary and liver function along with coagulation tests, comprehensive metabolic panel, and complete blood cell count with differential, should be acutely sent. In biliary obstruction, aspartate amniotransferase and alanine aminotransferase are variably increased. Alkaline phosphatase is increased and total bilirubin is also increased. In the presence of infection, white blood cells are increased and in liver disease transanamases are variably increased. Imaging tests follow, which include ultrasound, CT scan, or magnetic resonance cholangiopancreatography (MRCP) (**Fig. 7**).[81] Additional imaging occurs with treatment by endoscopic retrograde cholangiopancreatography (ERCP) or *percutaneous transhepatic cholangiography* (PTC) (discussed later).

Management

Management of biliary obstruction centers on urgent decompression of the biliary tract and restoration of bile drainage. Although this does not usually involve surgery per se, it is considered a surgical emergency. Relief of obstruction depends on the cause. In stone disease, ERCP is the first line and provides the opportunity for elimination of the impacted stone, imaging of the biliary tree, and drainage in one procedure.[82] In cases where ERCP is not possible or successful, drainage can be effected from above through PTC.[83,84] With drainage of the biliary tract, planning for repeat ERCP or operative exploration of the bile ducts can be undertaken in a nonemergent manner. In these cases, the bile duct is opened the obstruction relieved and closed over a T-tube. In cases where the biliary complication is associated with infection (cholangitis), emergent drainage is combined with resuscitation and broad-spectrum antibiotics (narrowed as culture results and sensitivities become available).[78,85,86] In cases of oncologic or anatomic obstruction, temporizing biliary drainage can be provided with PTC, thereby converting an emergent situation to an urgent or elective one, thereby allowing operative planning. Ultimately, the bile duct obstruction is resected or diverted, restoring biliary flow when the primary mass is addressed. In oncologic disease, the need for preoperative drainage is dependent on the degree of physiologic or infectious perturbation. In cases of stable physiology with no infection, the oncologic resection and reconstruction can often be the first intervention.

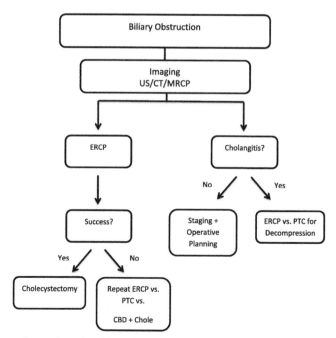

Fig. 7. Biliary obstruction algorithm. CBD, common bile duct exploration; Chole, cholecystectomy; US, ultrasound.

REFERENCES

1. Webb WA. Management of foreign bodies of the upper gastrointestinal tract: update. Gastrointest Endosc 1995;41(1):39–51.
2. Triadafilopoulos G, Roorda A, Akiyama J. Update on foreign bodies in the esophagus: diagnosis and management. Curr Gastroenterol Rep 2013;15(4):317.
3. Kirchner GI, Zuber-Jerger I, Endlicher E, et al. Causes of bolus impaction in the esophagus. Surg Endosc 2011;25(10):3170–4.
4. Sperry SL, Crockett SD, Miller CB, et al. Esophageal foreign-body impactions: epidemiology, time trends, and the impact of the increasing prevalence of eosinophilic esophagitis. Gastrointest Endosc 2011;74(5):985–91.
5. Crockett SD, Sperry SL, Miller CB, et al. Emergency care of esophageal foreign body impactions: timing, treatment modalities, and resource utilization. Dis Esophagus 2013;26(2):105–12.
6. Pinto A, Muzj C, Gagliardi N, et al. Role of imaging in the assessment of impacted foreign bodies in the hypopharynx and cervical esophagus. Semin Ultrasound CT MR 2012;33(5):463–70.
7. Eisen GM, Baron TH, Dominitz JA, et al. Guideline for the management of ingested foreign bodies. Gastrointest Endosc 2002;55(7):802–6.
8. Weant KA, Weant MP. Safety and efficacy of glucagon for the relief of acute esophageal food impaction. Am J Health Syst Pharm 2012;69(7):573–7.
9. Leopard D, Fishpool S, Winter S. The management of oesophageal soft food bolus obstruction: a systematic review. Ann R Coll Surg Engl 2011;93(6):441–4.
10. O'Keefe S, Rolniak S, Raina A, et al. Enteral feeding patients with gastric outlet obstruction. Nutr Clin Pract 2012;27(1):76–81.
11. Bawahab M, Mitchell P, Church N, et al. Management of acute paraesophageal hernia. Surg Endosc 2009;23(2):255–9.
12. Lappas JC, Reyes BL, Maglinte DD. Abdominal radiography findings in small-bowel obstruction: relevance to triage for additional diagnostic imaging. AJR Am J Roentgenol 2001;176(1):167–74.
13. Maglinte DD, Heitkamp DE, Howard TJ, et al. Current concepts in imaging of small bowel obstruction. Radiol Clin North Am 2003;41(2):263–83, vi.
14. Maglinte DD, Reyes BL, Harmon BH, et al. Reliability and role of plain film radiography and CT in the diagnosis of small-bowel obstruction. AJR Am J Roentgenol 1996;167(6):1451–5.
15. Maglinte DD, Kelvin FM, O'Connor K, et al. Current status of small bowel radiography. Abdom Imaging 1996;21(3):247–57.
16. Lee J. Bezoars and foreign bodies of the stomach. Gastrointest Endosc Clin N Am 1996;6(3):605–19.
17. Puri V, Lee RW, Amirlak BA, et al. Bouveret syndrome and gallstone ileus. Surg Laparosc Endosc Percutan Tech 2007;17(4):328–30.
18. Smith MT, Wong RK. Foreign bodies. Gastrointest Endosc Clin N Am 2007;17(2):361–82, vii.
19. Sevcik WE, Steiner IP. Acute gastric volvulus: case report and review of the literature. CJEM 1999;1(3):200–3.
20. Naim HJ, Smith R, Gorecki PJ. Emergent laparoscopic reduction of acute gastric volvulus with anterior gastropexy. Surg Laparosc Endosc Percutan Tech 2003;13(6):389–91.
21. Cherian PT, Cherian S, Singh P. Long-term follow-up of patients with gastric outlet obstruction related to peptic ulcer disease treated with endoscopic balloon dilatation and drug therapy. Gastrointest Endosc 2007;66(3):491–7.

22. Jeurnink SM, van Eijck CH, Steyerberg EW, et al. Stent versus gastrojejunostomy for the palliation of gastric outlet obstruction: a systematic review. BMC Gastroenterol 2007;7:18.
23. Jeurnink SM, Steyerberg EW, Hof G, et al. Gastrojejunostomy versus stent placement in patients with malignant gastric outlet obstruction: a comparison in 95 patients. J Surg Oncol 2007;96(5):389–96.
24. Rocha FG, Theman TA, Matros E, et al. Nonoperative management of patients with a diagnosis of high-grade small bowel obstruction by computed tomography. Arch Surg 2009;144(11):1000–4.
25. Ray NF, Denton WG, Thamer M, et al. Abdominal adhesiolysis: inpatient care and expenditures in the United States in 1994. J Am Coll Surg 1998;186(1):1–9.
26. Diaz JJ Jr, Bokhari F, Mowery NT, et al. Guidelines for management of small bowel obstruction. J Trauma 2008;64(6):1651–64.
27. Catena F, Di Saverio S, Kelly MD, et al. Bologna guidelines for diagnosis and management of adhesive small bowel obstruction (ASBO): 2010 evidence-based guidelines of the World Society of Emergency Surgery. World J Emerg Surg 2011;6:5.
28. Vallicelli C, Coccolini F, Catena F, et al. Small bowel emergency surgery: literature's review. World J Emerg Surg 2011;6(1):1.
29. Duron JJ, Silva NJ, du Montcel ST, et al. Adhesive postoperative small bowel obstruction: incidence and risk factors of recurrence after surgical treatment: a multicenter prospective study. Ann Surg 2006;244(5):750–7.
30. Sandrasegaran K, Maglinte DD, Howard TJ, et al. The multifaceted role of radiology in small bowel obstruction. Semin Ultrasound CT MR 2003;24(5):319–35.
31. Daneshmand S, Hedley CG, Stain SC. The utility and reliability of computed tomography scan in the diagnosis of small bowel obstruction. Am Surg 1999;65(10):922–6.
32. Taourel PG, Fabre JM, Pradel JA, et al. Value of CT in the diagnosis and management of patients with suspected acute small-bowel obstruction. AJR Am J Roentgenol 1995;165(5):1187–92.
33. Zalcman M, Sy M, Donckier V, et al. Helical CT signs in the diagnosis of intestinal ischemia in small-bowel obstruction. AJR Am J Roentgenol 2000;175(6):1601–7.
34. Tanaka S, Yamamoto T, Kubota D, et al. Predictive factors for surgical indication in adhesive small bowel obstruction. Am J Surg 2008;196(1):23–7.
35. Lazarus DE, Slywotsky C, Bennett GL, et al. Frequency and relevance of the "small-bowel feces" sign on CT in patients with small-bowel obstruction. AJR Am J Roentgenol 2004;183(5):1361–6.
36. Gollub MJ, Yoon S, Smith LM, et al. Does the CT whirl sign really predict small bowel volvulus?: experience in an oncologic population. J Comput Assist Tomogr 2006;30(1):25–32.
37. Murray MJ, Gonze MD, Nowak LR, et al. Serum D(-)-lactate levels as an aid to diagnosing acute intestinal ischemia. Am J Surg 1994;167(6):575–8.
38. Poeze M, Froon AH, Greve JW, et al. D-lactate as an early marker of intestinal ischaemia after ruptured abdominal aortic aneurysm repair. Br J Surg 1998;85(9):1221–4.
39. Evennett NJ, Petrov MS, Mittal A, et al. Systematic review and pooled estimates for the diagnostic accuracy of serological markers for intestinal ischemia. World J Surg 2009;33(7):1374–83.
40. Cosse C, Regimbeau JM, Fuks D, et al. Serum procalcitonin for predicting the failure of conservative management and the need for bowel resection in patients with small bowel obstruction. J Am Coll Surg 2013;216(5):997–1004.

41. Foster NM, McGory ML, Zingmond DS, et al. Small bowel obstruction: a population-based appraisal. J Am Coll Surg 2006;203(2):170–6.
42. Zielinski MD, Eiken PW, Bannon MP, et al. Small bowel obstruction-who needs an operation? A multivariate prediction model. World J Surg 2010;34(5):910–9.
43. Hayanga AJ, Bass-Wilkins K, Bulkley GB. Current management of small-bowel obstruction. Adv Surg 2005;39:1–33.
44. Li MZ, Lian L, Xiao LB, et al. Laparoscopic versus open adhesiolysis in patients with adhesive small bowel obstruction: a systematic review and meta-analysis. Am J Surg 2012;204(5):779–86.
45. Mancini GJ, Petroski GF, Lin WC, et al. Nationwide impact of laparoscopic lysis of adhesions in the management of intestinal obstruction in the US. J Am Coll Surg 2008;207(4):520–6.
46. Suter M, Zermatten P, Halkic N, et al. Laparoscopic management of mechanical small bowel obstruction: are there predictors of success or failure? Surg Endosc 2000;14(5):478–83.
47. Khaikin M, Schneidereit N, Cera S, et al. Laparoscopic vs. open surgery for acute adhesive small-bowel obstruction: patients' outcome and cost-effectiveness. Surg Endosc 2007;21(5):742–6.
48. O'Connor DB, Winter DC. The role of laparoscopy in the management of acute small-bowel obstruction: a review of over 2,000 cases. Surg Endosc 2012;26(1):12–7.
49. Cirocchi R, Abraha I, Farinella E, et al. Laparoscopic versus open surgery in small bowel obstruction. Cochrane Database Syst Rev 2010;(2):CD007511.
50. Ghosheh B, Salameh JR. Laparoscopic approach to acute small bowel obstruction: review of 1061 cases. Surg Endosc 2007;21(11):1945–9.
51. Assalia A, Schein M, Kopelman D, et al. Therapeutic effect of oral Gastrografin in adhesive, partial small-bowel obstruction: a prospective randomized trial. Surgery 1994;115(4):433–7.
52. Biondo S, Pares D, Mora L, et al. Randomized clinical study of Gastrografin administration in patients with adhesive small bowel obstruction. Br J Surg 2003;90(5):542–6.
53. Choi HK, Chu KW, Law WL. Therapeutic value of gastrografin in adhesive small bowel obstruction after unsuccessful conservative treatment: a prospective randomized trial. Ann Surg 2002;236(1):1–6.
54. Blackmon S, Lucius C, Wilson JP, et al. The use of water-soluble contrast in evaluating clinically equivocal small bowel obstruction. Am Surg 2000;66(3):238–42 [discussion: 242–4].
55. Bickell NA, Federman AD, Aufses AH Jr. Influence of time on risk of bowel resection in complete small bowel obstruction. J Am Coll Surg 2005;201(6):847–54.
56. Fevang BT, Jensen D, Svanes K, et al. Early operation or conservative management of patients with small bowel obstruction? Eur J Surg 2002;168(8–9):475–81.
57. Schraufnagel D, Rajaee S, Millham FH. How many sunsets? Timing of surgery in adhesive small bowel obstruction: a study of the Nationwide Inpatient Sample. J Trauma Acute Care Surg 2013;74(1):181–7 [discussion: 187–9].
58. Ellozy SH, Harris MT, Bauer JJ, et al. Early postoperative small-bowel obstruction: a prospective evaluation in 242 consecutive abdominal operations. Dis Colon Rectum 2002;45(9):1214–7.
59. Pickleman J, Lee RM. The management of patients with suspected early postoperative small bowel obstruction. Ann Surg 1989;210(2):216–9.

60. Fraser SA, Shrier I, Miller G, et al. Immediate postlaparotomy small bowel obstruction: a 16-year retrospective analysis. Am Surg 2002;68(9):780–2.
61. Miller G, Boman J, Shrier I, et al. Readmission for small-bowel obstruction in the early postoperative period: etiology and outcome. Can J Surg 2002;45(4): 255–8.
62. Carmichael JC, Mills S. Reoperation for small bowel obstruction–how critical is the timing? Clin Colon Rectal Surg 2006;19(4):181–7.
63. Lopez-Kostner F, Hool GR, Lavery IC. Management and causes of acute large-bowel obstruction. Surg Clin North Am 1997;77(6):1265–90.
64. Ballantyne GH, Brandner MD, Beart RW Jr, et al. Volvulus of the colon. Incidence and mortality. Ann Surg 1985;202(1):83–92.
65. Mulas C, Bruna M, Garcia-Armengol J, et al. Management of colonic volvulus. Experience in 75 patients. Rev Esp Enferm Dig 2010;102(4):239–48.
66. Friedman JD, Odland MD, Bubrick MP. Experience with colonic volvulus. Dis Colon Rectum 1989;32(5):409–16.
67. Young-Fadok TM, Roberts PL, Spencer MP, et al. Colonic diverticular disease. Curr Probl Surg 2000;37(7):457–514.
68. Etzioni DA, Mack TM, Beart RW Jr, et al. Diverticulitis in the United States: 1998-2005: changing patterns of disease and treatment. Ann Surg 2009;249(2): 210–7.
69. Simpson J, Spiller R. Colonic diverticular disease. Clin Evid 2004;(12):599–609.
70. Tursi A. Is elective surgery mandatory after an attack of acute colonic diverticulitis? Some remarks about the new pathophysiology of the diverticular disease. Dis Colon Rectum 2009;52(1):168–9.
71. Trompetas V. Emergency management of malignant acute left-sided colonic obstruction. Ann R Coll Surg Engl 2008;90(3):181–6.
72. Gainant A. Emergency management of acute colonic cancer obstruction. J Visc Surg 2012;149(1):e3–10.
73. Feo L, Schaffzin DM. Colonic stents: the modern treatment of colonic obstruction. Adv Ther 2011;28(2):73–86.
74. Grossman EB, Schattner MA, Dimaio CJ, et al. Endoscopic management of complete colonic obstruction. J Interv Gastroenterol 2011;1(4):179–81.
75. Khan MI, Claydon A. Colonic self-expanding metal stents (SEMS) in acute large bowel obstruction. N Z Med J 2011;124(1345):57–63.
76. Song LM, Baron TH. Stenting for acute malignant colonic obstruction: a bridge to nowhere? Lancet Oncol 2011;12(4):314–5.
77. Oren D, Atamanalp SS, Aydinli B, et al. An algorithm for the management of sigmoid colon volvulus and the safety of primary resection: experience with 827 cases. Dis Colon Rectum 2007;50(4):489–97.
78. Attasaranya S, Fogel EL, Lehman GA. Choledocholithiasis, ascending cholangitis, and gallstone pancreatitis. Med Clin North Am 2008;92(4):925–60, x.
79. Remes-Troche JM, Perez-Martinez C, Rembis V, et al. Surgical treatment of colonic volvulus. 10-year experience at the Instituto Nacional de la Nutricion Salvador Zubiran [in Spanish]. Rev Gastroenterol Mex 1997;62(4):276–80.
80. Geer DA, Arnaud G, Beitler A, et al. Colonic volvulus. The Army Medical Center experience 1983-1987. Am Surg 1991;57(5):295–300.
81. Chan YL, Chan AC, Lam WW, et al. Choledocholithiasis: comparison of MR cholangiography and endoscopic retrograde cholangiography. Radiology 1996; 200(1):85–9.
82. Adler DG, Baron TH, Davila RE, et al. ASGE guideline: the role of ERCP in diseases of the biliary tract and the pancreas. Gastrointest Endosc 2005;62(1):1–8.

83. Tsuyuguchi T, Takada T, Miyazaki M, et al. Stenting and interventional radiology for obstructive jaundice in patients with unresectable biliary tract carcinomas. J Hepatobiliary Pancreat Surg 2008;15(1):69–73.

84. Mueller PR. Interventional radiology of the biliary tract: a decade of progress. Radiology 1988;168(2):328–30.

85. Mosler P. Diagnosis and management of acute cholangitis. Curr Gastroenterol Rep 2011;13(2):166–72.

86. Gallix BP, Aufort S, Pierredon MA, et al. Acute cholangitis: imaging diagnosis and management [in French]. J Radiol 2006;87(4 Pt 2):430–40.

Hernia Emergencies

D. Dante Yeh, MD[a],*, Hasan B. Alam, MD[b]

KEYWORDS

- Hernia • Emergencies • Acute care surgery

KEY POINTS

- Hernia emergencies are commonly encountered by the acute care surgeon.
- Although the location and contents may vary, the basic principles are constant: address the life-threatening problem first, then perform the safest and most durable hernia repair possible.
- Mesh reinforcement provides the most durable long-term results.
- Underlay positioning is associated with the best outcomes.
- Components separation is a useful technique to achieve tension-free primary fascial reapproximation.
- The choice of mesh is dictated by the degree of contamination.
- Internal herniation is rare, and preoperative diagnosis remains difficult.
- In all hernia emergencies, morbidity is high, and postoperative wound complications should be anticipated.

INCARCERATED INGUINAL AND FEMORAL HERNIAS
Definitions

A hernia is a weakness or disruption of the fibromuscular tissues through which an internal organ (or part of the organ) protrudes or slides through. Collectively, inguinal and femoral hernias are often lumped together into groin hernias. Inguinal hernias can be indirect or direct. Indirect hernia protrudes through the internal inguinal ring, which is an opening in the transversalis fascia, located laterally to the inferior epigastric artery. Direct inguinal hernia, on the other hand, comes out through the Hesselbach triangle (bounded laterally by the inferior epigastric vessels, medially by the lateral border of the rectus muscle, and inferiorly by the inguinal ligament). Femoral hernias protrude through the femoral canal, which is located below the inguinal ligament on the lateral aspect of the pubic tubercle. It is bounded by the inguinal ligament anteriorly, pectineal ligament posteriorly, lacunar ligament medially, and the femoral vein laterally. This is a tight opening bordered by sturdy ligaments, which makes it more susceptible

[a] Department of Surgery, Massachusetts General Hospital, Harvard Medical School, 165 Cambridge Street, Suite 810, Boston, MA 02114, USA; [b] Department of Surgery, University of Michigan Health System, 1500 East Medical Center Drive, Ann Arbor, MI 48109, USA
* Corresponding author.
E-mail address: DYEH2@PARTNERS.ORG

Surg Clin N Am 94 (2014) 97–130
http://dx.doi.org/10.1016/j.suc.2013.10.009
0039-6109/14/$ – see front matter © 2014 Elsevier Inc. All rights reserved.
surgical.theclinics.com

to strangulation. It is also located rather deep, which obscures the physical examination and often delays the diagnosis.

The following terms are important to clarify when discussing hernias: (1) reducible, which refers to a hernia that can go back into the body cavity easily (either manually or spontaneously); (2) irreducible/incarcerated, which refers to a hernia that cannot be reduced; it does not automatically mean that the hernia is strangulated or that obstruction is occurring (although both are possible); and (3) strangulated, which refers to a hernia in which the blood supply to the incarcerated contents is compromised.

Epidemiology

Hernias are among the oldest recorded afflictions of humans, and inguinal hernia repair is one of the most common general surgical procedures.[1] Inguinal hernias comprise 70% to 75% of all abdominal wall hernias and are more common in men, whereas femoral hernias account for less than 5% and are more common in women.[2,3] Overall, 96% of groin hernias are inguinal and 4% are femoral. These hernias are more common in men. The lifetime risk of developing a groin hernia is 25% in men, but less than 5% in women. Men are also 20-fold more likely to need a hernia repair.

When to Repair?

Surgery remains the only effective treatment, but the optimal timing and method of repair remain controversial. Although strangulation rates of 3% at 3 months have been reported by some investigators,[4] the largest prospective randomized trial (n = 720) of (watchful waiting) men with minimally symptomatic inguinal hernias showed that watchful waiting is safe.[5] Frequency of strangulation was only 2.4% in patients followed up for as long as 11.5 years. Long-term follow-up shows that more than two-thirds of men using a strategy of watchful waiting cross over to surgical repair, with pain being the most common reasons. This risk of crossover is higher in patients older than 65 years.[6] Once an inguinal hernia becomes symptomatic, surgical repair is clearly indicated. Femoral hernias are more likely to present with strangulation and require emergency surgery[7] and are thus repaired even when asymptomatic. Because this article focuses on incarcerated hernias, nonoperative options are not discussed.

How to Repair?

Open versus laparoscopic

The laparoscopic approach has gained popularity for the repair of nonincarcerated groin hernias, but randomized trials have shown that this approach has a higher recurrence rate, more serious complications, requires a substantial learning curve, and is not cost-effective.[8,9] A large European study showed that laparoscopic repair was no better than open, with a higher chance of technical errors.[10] In expert hands it remains an attractive option, and often its selection for elective repairs is driven by patient demand. However, once the hernia has become incarcerated, an open approach is the safest, because it allows for proper evaluation of the hernia contents, safe reduction, resection (if needed), and a secure repair.

Mesh versus primary

In recent years, Lichtenstein tension-free mesh-based repair has become the criterion standard for elective hernia repair.[11] Numerous permanent meshes are available, with no convincing data establishing the superiority of any particular brand/mesh type. In the setting of bowel incarceration, if there is no ischemia and no need for resection, use of permanent mesh is still relatively safe.[12,13] However, implantation of permanent synthetic mesh in the setting of bowel ischemia/resection can lead to an unacceptably high risk of mesh infection and long-term complications. Biological meshes have been shown to be resistant to infections, but their use in contaminated fields is associated with poor long-term durability of the repair.[14] Because fixing the acute problem is a higher priority than the long-term durability of the repair, our preference is to either use a biological mesh or perform a traditional mesh-free tissue repair (eg, Bassini, McVay, or Shouldice repairs). Hernia recurrence rates are no doubt higher with this approach, but at the time of recurrence, an elective repair with a permanent mesh repair can be performed more safely.

Perioperative Decision Making

Should a painful hernia be reduced before surgery?

A strangulated hernia should not be reduced preoperatively. Doing so results in pushing a loop of dead/threatened bowel into the peritoneal cavity and converts a localized process into diffuse peritonitis. Also, this procedure forces the surgeon to perform laparoscopy/laparotomy to evaluate the bowel and to decrease the chances of delayed complications (eg, perforation of ischemic bowel or ischemic stricture). The safest approach is to immediately take the patient to the operating room for a local exploration via a groin incision (but be ready for laparotomy). The surgeon must ensure the viability of the bowel in the sac before it is reduced into the peritoneal cavity. Should an incarcerated hernia be managed in a similar fashion? In an acutely incarcerated hernia that shows no signs of impending ischemia (eg, tenderness, increased white blood cell count, fever, skin changes), an attempt at reduction is not unreasonable. This strategy can prevent its progression to strangulation and allow a more elective operation. Our preference in such cases is to repair the hernia during the same hospital admission, typically after a 12-hour to 24-hour period of observation (after reduction). This period of observation should identify the small subset of patients in whom the reduced bowel is nonviable. At the same time, vigorous attempts to reduce an incarcerated hernia, especially if tender or incarcerated for more than a short period, are misguided. The safest approach is to take such a patient to the operating room for examination of hernia sac contents and careful reduction under general anesthesia after ensuring bowel viability.

Radiographic workup

Incarcerated or strangulated inguinal hernias do not require any radiographic workup unless the diagnosis is in doubt (eg, unreliable examination in an obese patient), or the contribution of hernia to the symptoms is unclear (eg, possible epididymitis/orchitis/torsion in a patient with hernia). Radiographic studies can delay the definitive operative intervention and worsen the outcomes. Femoral hernias are notoriously difficult to appreciate on physical examination and are often discovered on radiologic studies (computed tomography [CT] or ultrasonography).

Unable to reduce- what now?

Infrequently, the hernia neck is too tight (or sac too large) to permit open intraoperative reduction, even under general anesthesia. Opening the sac and putting the patient in a steep Trendelenburg position helps. If this strategy is unsuccessful, then the surgeon should not hesitate to enlarge the hernia defect. A solid familiarity with the anatomic boundaries of the defect is essential to avoid causing iatrogenic injury to critical adjacent structures. In case of indirect inguinal hernia, the internal oblique/conjoint fibers can be incised in an upward direction. Direct hernias rarely pose this problem but can be treated the same as indirect hernia. Femoral hernias are more challenging. A small incision to partially divide the inguinal ligament anteriorly should suffice. Alternatively, the lacunar ligament can be divided medially (be aware of an aberrant obturator artery, which can pass in the anterior margin of the lucanar ligament in up to 30%). In very large, chronic hernias, reduction may be challenging because of loss of domain, but they rarely need emergent surgery. Despite being nonreducible, strangulation is a rare event in these giant hernias.

Loop of dead bowel in the hernia: what next?

If dead bowel is found on opening the hernia sac, the next step depends on the quality of the surgical exposure. If the hernia defect can be enlarged sufficiently to permit safe resection and anastomosis of the bowel, then performing the procedure through the groin incision is reasonable. After reducing the anastomosed bowel back into the abdomen, the hernia defect can be repaired either with a biological mesh or primary tissue approximation. However, there should be a low threshold to convert the operation into a laparotomy if better exposure is required for the bowel resection, or if the extent of the threatened bowel is unclear. The hernia can then be fixed either from inside the abdomen or through the groin incision.

Other Issues

Bilateral hernias

There seems to be increasing consensus that for elective repair of bilateral symptomatic hernias[15] or recurrent hernias, the laparoscopic approach is appropriate. However, for an emergent situation, our recommendation is to repair the incarcerated/strangulated hernia using an open approach, without worrying about the contralateral hernia. Once the patient has recovered from the acute episode, an elective repair of the other side can be performed either open or laparoscopically.

Cancer

Rarely, incarcerated bowel is found to have a mass that might be malignant. In such cases, basic surgical oncology principles apply. An appropriate cancer resection of the bowel, including adequate mesentery/lymph nodes, should be performed. This situation invariably requires converting the procedure to a standard laparotomy.

INCARCERATED UMBILICAL/INCISIONAL/ABDOMINAL WALL HERNIA

Epidemiology

Ventral hernias (VH) are a family of hernias involving the anterior abdominal wall. They are diagnosed on physical examination by the presence of a bulge and often come to the patient's attention because of visual appearance, discomfort, pain, intestinal obstruction, or intestinal infarction. Some VH can enlarge to such an extent that the bulk of abdominal contents come to reside within the hernia sac and it becomes physically impossible to reduce back into the abdominal cavity proper. This scenario is referred to as loss of domain.

The natural history of VH is to progressively enlarge over time. Emergency repair, required in up to 20% of VH, is naturally associated with poorer outcomes, and elective repair is generally recommended on diagnosis.[16] Incarceration with strangulation is less common in cases with a very small hernia neck (<1 cm) or very large hernia neck (where bowel loops can easily move in and out of the sac without restriction). VH can be broadly classified into congenital and acquired causes; however, the principles of treatment are similar for all hernia emergencies of the abdominal wall.

Congenital

Epigastric

Located between the xiphoid process and umbilicus, epigastric hernias occur in approximately 3% to 5% of the population and are more common in men.[17] Most are small (1 cm), and only 50% are symptomatic. Twenty percent are multiple. Hernia contents are usually preperitoneal fat, and it is rare that bowel becomes incarcerated in congenital epigastric hernias.

Umbilical

As the name implies, umbilical hernias occur in the periumbilical region. Most congenital umbilical hernias close spontaneously by the age of 5 years, and most umbilical hernias encountered in adults are acquired.

Hypogastric

Hypogastric hernias occur below the umbilicus and rarely develop spontaneously.

Acquired

Incisional

Most abdominal wall hernias are acquired postoperatively through the surgical incision, although there are some rare acquired hernias, which are discussed later. Incisional hernias are estimated to occur after 10% to 30% of laparotomies,[18–20] and almost 150,000 incisional hernia repairs are performed each year in the United States. Risk factors for postoperative incisional hernia development include wound infection, obesity, male gender, older age, smoking, steroid use, chemotherapy, connective tissue diseases, and malnutrition.[21] Less well-studied factors include closure technique (suture material, continuous vs interrupted) and incision type. The highest incidence occurs after midline incisions, with lower incidence after transverse and paramedian incisions.[22] Almost 20% of incisional hernias are incarcerated or strangulated on initial presentation, and these emergent repairs are associated with worse outcomes.[23,24]

Although less common, incisional hernia can also occur after laparoscopic operations, with the reported incidence between 0.6% and 2.8%. Most trocar-site hernias occur through ports more than 10 mm in the umbilicus, and it is strongly recommended to primarily close these trocar sites at the completion of laparoscopic surgery.[25]

Umbilical

Acquired umbilical hernias are believed to develop secondary to increased intra-abdominal pressure and are associated with conditions such as pregnancy, cirrhosis with ascites, obesity, and large abdominal tumors. They are more common in women, and it is estimated that only 5% require emergent repair.[26]

Umbilical hernia develops in 20% of patients with liver cirrhosis, which is significantly increased above the 2% incidence seen in the general population.[27,28] If ascites is present, this incidence increases further to 40%.[29] Reasons for this increased incidence include increased intra-abdominal pressure secondary to ascites, malnutrition, and dilation of the recanalized umbilical vein. These dilated umbilical veins (secondary to portosystemic collateral flow) can make the dissection treacherous (**Fig. 1**). The risk of precipitating esophageal variceal bleeding after umbilical hernia repair is controversial, and claims of an association have not been confirmed.[30–32]

Historically, surgeons were reluctant to repair these hernias electively, because early reports documented perioperative mortality as high as 16% to 31%.[30,31] However, recent series have shown that, with modern perioperative care, mortality after elective umbilical hernia repair does not differ between cirrhotics and noncirrhotics. It is recommended to repair umbilical hernias electively in cirrhotic patients, because emergency operation is significantly more morbid than elective repair.[33,34]

Reasons for emergency repair include bowel incarceration, skin ulceration/erosion with leakage of ascites, and bowel evisceration.[35] Patients usually report progressive

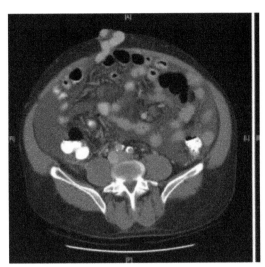

Fig. 1. Dilated umbilical veins. (*From* Shlomovitz E, Quan D, Etemad-Rezai R, et al. Association of recanalization of the left umbilical vein with umbilical hernia in patients with liver disease. Liver Transpl 2005;11(10):1298–9; with permission.)

enlargement, although 1 rare presentation is sudden incarceration after ascites decompression via paracentesis.[36,37] history of antecedent skin ulceration is elicited in most patients (80%) presenting with ruptured spontaneous paracentesis, and this finding should be considered an indication for urgent repair, because mortality after spontaneous rupture is up to 30%.[28,38] Depending on the degree of physiologic derangement, the repair may be delayed if resuscitation and metabolic correction are required. In the interim, the hernia should be covered with a sterile occlusive dressing and the patient treated with antibiotics. Nonsurgical management of ruptured umbilical hernia is associated with mortality up to 88%.[38]

The strongest factor influencing umbilical hernia recurrence after repair in cirrhotic patients is the presence of ascites.[39] Recurrence rate after primary repair in cirrhotic patients with ascites is as high as 73%.[31,39] Multiple adjuncts have been described, including medical diuretic therapy, peritoneovenous shunting,[40,41] transjugular intrahepatic portosystemic shunting,[28,42,43] and temporary peritoneal dialysis catheter placement.[44] Our preference is to use closed-suction drainage combined with skin adhesive 2-octyl cyanoacrylate (Ethicon) reinforcement of the skin closure for a watertight seal. The optimal duration of postoperative ascites drainage is unknown, and the decision to remove the drain should be considered on a case-by-case basis.

Anatomy of the Anterior Abdominal Wall

A thorough understanding of the musculature of the anterior abdominal wall is required to effectively repair herniation in this body region (**Fig. 2**). Laterally, from most superficial to deep, the 3 muscles are the external oblique, internal oblique, and transversus abdominis. Medially, a paired longitudinal muscle, the rectus abdominis, is enveloped by a strong fascial sheath comprising the fused aponeurotic extensions of the aforementioned lateral muscles. The right and left rectus sheath are fused at the midline structure, the linea alba.

The umbilicus is the obliterated remnant of the umbilical cord, and is marked by the confluence of adult remnants of fetal circulation: the ligamentum teres, the medial umbilical folds, and the median umbilical ligament.

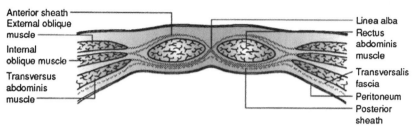

Fig. 2. Layers of the anterior abdominal wall. (*From* Fitzgibbons RC Jr, S, Quinn TH. Abdominal wall hernias. In: Mulholland KD, Lillimoe KD, Doherty GM, et al, editors. Greenfield's surgery: scientific principles and practice. New York: Wolters Kluwer/Lippincott Williams & Wilkins; 2011. p. 1163; with permission.)

An important anatomic landmark is the arcuate line, located a few centimeters caudal to the umbilicus. Below this boundary, the posterior rectus sheath is absent, and all aponeurotic layers pass anterior to the rectus muscle.

Mesh options

An in-depth description and comparison of all available meshes is beyond the scope of this review. The choice of a particular brand is commonly dictated by hospital availability and surgeon familiarity. With a confusing array of options, it is helpful to broadly categorize meshes according to their basic characteristics. The main distinction is between synthetic and biological material.

Permanent synthetic The term prosthetic applies to a mesh composed of a permanent, synthetic material, usually polypropylene, polyester, or expanded polytetrafluoroethylene. Prosthetics are available in a variety of weights and pore sizes, allowing for varying rates of native fibroblast ingrowth and incorporation into the host tissue. Only certain prosthetic meshes with a smooth microporous surface are appropriate for intraperitoneal placement (**Table 1**). Direct contact between macroporous meshes and bowel is associated with unacceptably high rates of erosion or fistulization. If there is no risk of bowel contact, microporous mesh is not recommended, because the tight weave prevents adequate vascular ingrowth (but still allowing bacterial infiltration), increasing the risk of infection, encapsulation, and seroma formation.

Absorbable Absorbable synthetic meshes such as polyglactin (Ethicon) are not durable enough for definitive repair but may be considered in a grossly infected wound, in which permanent prosthesis implantation is contraindicated and an expensive biological graft is quickly digested by the high collagenase activity present in the wound.

Table 1	
Prosthetic mesh options	
Extraperitoneal Only	**Intra-abdominal**
Prolene (Ethicon)	DualMesh, DualMesh Plus (W. L. Gore)
Marlex (Bard)	Dulex (Bard/Davol)
Ultrapro (Ethicon)	Composix (Bard/Davol)
ProLite (Atrium)	Sepramesh (Genzyme)
TiMesh (Biomet)	Proceed (Ethicon)
Parietex (Covidien)	C-Qur (Atrium)
Mersilene (Ethicon)	Parietex Composite (Covidien)
MotifMesh (Proxy Biomedical)	

Biological Biological grafts have been available for VH repair since 2003 and are derived from human, porcine, and bovine tissue (dermis, small intestine, or pericardium). Not only can they serve initially as a mechanical bridge but they may also function as a scaffold during subsequent tissue remodeling, when the host's native tissue digests and replaces the graft with native collagen. Postprocurement processing is performed to remove cellular material, preventing a foreign body response by the host, and leaving behind the collagen/elastin matrix. In addition, some grafts are treated with cross-linking to prolong the time required by the host to integrate the graft.[45] Because of infiltration by host immune cells and abundant vascularity secondary to angiogenesis, it is thought that biological grafts have enhanced ability to resist infection, making them a preferred choice for use in contaminated fields (**Box 1**).

Bioprosthesis durability in hernia repair is questionable, with recurrence rates as high as 80% reported when used without fascial support.[46–48]

Although the use of biological grafts is favored in heavily contaminated operative fields, their cost-effectiveness in clean and minimally contaminated cases remains to be determined, because these grafts are, on average, 10 times more expensive than prosthetic meshes. A recent systematic review reported wound complication rates of 26.2% and a recurrence rate of 15.7%, comparable with results with synthetic meshes.[49] Comparisons between biological grafts suggest that human-derived grafts are more likely to stretch and result in hernia recurrence but less likely to become infected and require explantation.[50,51]

In a study of single-stage VH bioprosthetic repairs in contaminated or infected fields, Rosen and colleagues[14] reported a 31% hernia recurrence rate at a mean follow-up of 21 months. However, only a small percentage of these patients required reoperation (5.5% of the original cohort). Postoperative wound complications occurred in one-half of patients. Despite manufacturer claims and general support

---

Box 1
Biological graft options

Human dermis

  Alloderm (LifeCell)

  Allomax (Bard/Davol)

  Flex HD (MTF)

Porcine dermis

  Permacol (TSL)

  Collamend (Bard/Davol)

  Strattice (LifeCell)

  XenMatrix (Brennan Medical)

Porcine small intestine

  Surgisis (Cook)

Fetal bovine dermis

  Surgimend (TEI Bioscience)

Bovine pericardium

  Tutopatch (Tutogen)

  Veritas (Synovis)

in review articles, the bulk of the primary literature supporting the use of biological grafts for VH repair in contaminated fields consists of case series and case reports (the lowest level of evidence), and that their use in these scenarios has not been cleared or approved by the US Food and Drug Administration.[52]

Components separation

Components separation (CS) or separation of parts, first described by Ramirez and colleagues[53] in 1990, is a technique designed to enlarge the abdominal cavity by separating the layers of muscle and disconnecting them from their fascial attachments, allowing for individual translation and maximal expansion. It entails a relaxing incision through the external oblique aponeurosis 2 cm lateral to the rectus sheath and dissection in the plane between the external oblique and internal oblique muscles, as well as dissection and release of the rectus abdominis from the posterior rectus sheath (**Fig. 3**). This dissection is carried superiorly to the costal margin and inferiorly down to the inguinal ligament. Some investigators recommend extending the superior aspect 5 cm above the costal margin to decrease the risk of epigastric recurrence, the most common site of recurrence.[54]

CS can provide up to 10 cm of unilateral medial advancement of the fascial edge (20 cm if performed bilaterally) and is a useful technique to achieve primary fascial closure in cases of massive VH. The CS procedure is accompanied with its own set of complications, which are more common in the setting of contamination.[55] Because of the extensive dissection required, the patient is left with large skin flaps; wound complications such as surgical site infection and seroma/hematoma are common.[54,56]

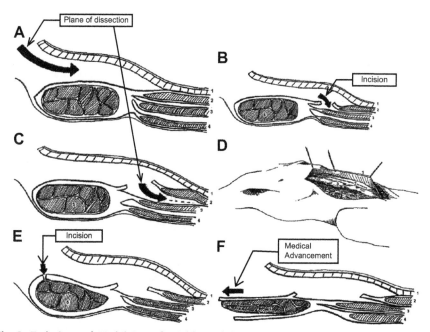

Fig. 3. Technique of CS. (*A*) Suprafascial lateral dissection (*B*) External oblique aponeurosis incision, (*C*) Dissection deep to external oblique muscle, (*D*) Medical traction, (*E*) Rectus sheath incision, (*F*) Additional Medical Advancement. (*From* de Vries Reilingh TS, van Goor H, Rosman C, et al. "Components separation technique" for the repair of large abdominal wall hernias. J Am Coll Surg 2003;196(1):32–7; with permission.)

A more serious complication is ischemia and necrosis of the flaps, occurring in up to 6%. When used alone without mesh reinforcement, CS is associated with recurrence rates as high as 53%.[54,57]

To address these complications, several modifications to the technique have been developed:

1. Mesh reinforcement: to decrease the incidence of hernia recurrence, the use of both prosthetic and biological prosthesis reinforcement of the primary fascial closure has been described in both onlay, inlay, and underlay configurations. A sandwich technique using both underlay and onlay reinforcement has been reported to have a recurrence rate of only 3.9%.[56] The Ventral Hernia Working Group (VHWG) recommends reinforcement of CS closure.[58]
2. Rectus abdominis muscle plication: a recent report described 13 patients who underwent rectus plication (similar to abdominoplasty or tummy tuck) as tissue reinforcement of CS. The investigators contend that this technique decreases tension along the line of closure, provides an additional barrier of tissue atop the hernia closure, and does not require additional dissection. With only 1 recurrence over a mean follow-up of 24 months, this technique may be a more cost-effective method of reinforcement than prosthesis, but more studies are required before strong recommendations can be made.[59]
3. Minimally invasive CS: using 2-cm to 3-cm incisions and laparoscopic equipment, several investigators have reported comparable operative times and hospital length of stay, with the benefit of significantly decreased wound complications when compared with traditional CS (**Fig. 4**).[60–62] One disadvantage to this method is that the degree of abdominal wall advancement is only 86% of that achievable by open CS, likely because of tethering of the abdominal wall muscles to the overlying tissue.[63]
4. Posterior CS: in this variation, only the posterior component of the original Ramirez technique is performed. The posterior rectus sheath is incised 1 to 2 cm lateral to the midline, and the rectus abdominis muscle is dissected free from the sheath.[64]

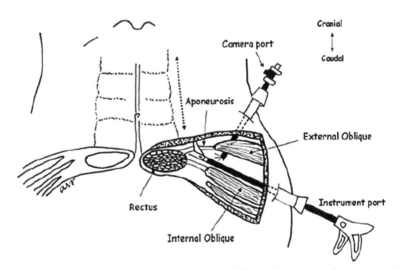

Fig. 4. Endoscopic CS. (*From* Rosen MJ, Jin J, McGee MF, et al. Laparoscopic component separation in the single-stage treatment of infected abdominal wall prosthetic removal. Hernia 2007;11(5):435–40; with permission.)

The lateral posterior rectus sheath (ie, the posterior leaflet of the internal oblique aponeurosis) is subsequently incised, allowing the surgeon to access the plane between the internal oblique muscle and the transversus abdominis muscle (**Fig. 5**). This technique allows for not only medial advancement of the abdominal wall musculature but also a plane for the placement of an underlay mesh reinforcement. The advantage of this technique is that it avoids the need for an extensive subcutaneous dissection and its attendant wound complications; however, the extent of medial advancement afforded is less than that of external oblique release.[65,66]

After dissection of the subcutaneous plane, superficial seroma is near universal, and it is customary to leave closed-suction drains until the output is less than 30 mL/d for 2 consecutive days. This process may take up to 4 weeks. Prolonged antibiotic prophylaxis is not indicated.

Intraoperative decision making
Intraoperative decision making during emergency hernia repair should proceed in a logical fashion. First and foremost, the problem necessitating emergent operation should be addressed. The 2 most common reasons are complete bowel obstruction and incarceration with strangulation. After entering the abdomen (usually through the midline or previous incision), the hernia sac is reduced, enlarging the constricting ring as necessary. Any frankly necrotic segments of intestine should be resected, and marginal-appearing segments may be left in situ for later reassessment. If the patient is severely physiologically compromised, it may be prudent to apply the damage control principles of performing the minimum necessary to sustain life (arrest hemorrhage and control contamination), leaving the bowel in discontinuity and returning for definitive repair under more favorable conditions after correction of metabolic derangements.

Only after life-threatening issues have been fixed should the surgeon attempt hernia repair. With the understanding that emergent hernia operations present less than ideal circumstances, the surgeon should perform the safest and most durable repair possible. A single-stage repair should be attempted, unless massive loss of domain precludes closure and thus a staged repair is necessary.

Umbilical
If the fascial defect is less than 3 cm, primary repair alone is acceptable. For the better part of the twentieth century, umbilical hernia was repaired according to the vest-over-pants overlap technique described by Mayo in 1901.[67] However, recurrences up to 54% have been reported with the Mayo repair, and this repair method has been largely abandoned.[68,69] Data from randomized trials show that recurrence of umbilical hernia is significantly lower (as low as 1%) with tension-free mesh repair when compared with primary fascial repair.[70,71] In the absence of contraindications, mesh prosthetic reinforcement is strongly recommended for defects larger than 3 cm. Some investigators have even reported superior outcomes with mesh reinforcement for defects smaller

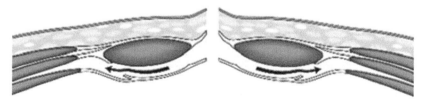

Fig. 5. Technique of posterior CS. (*From* Carbonell AM, Cobb WS, Chen SM. Posterior components separation during retromuscular hernia repair. Hernia 2008;12(4):359–62; with permission.)

than 3 cm.[70] Options for prosthetic mesh closure include plug reinforcement, sheet underlay, and Prolene hernia system (PHS).[72,73]

Incisional

For defects larger than 3 cm, every attempt should be made to achieve midline approximation of the rectus abdominis for primary fascial closure, using CS techniques if necessary.[58] However, because of the high recurrence rate of primary fascial repair alone (50%), mesh reinforcement should be considered in all circumstances.[21] Strong long-term, high-quality evidence supports the routine use of mesh reinforcement for repair of incisional hernias.[74–76] The American Hernia Society declares that the use of mesh represents the current standard of care for incisional hernia repair, and the VHWG makes a strong recommendation for routine mesh reinforcement of all incisional VH repairs.[58,77] The choice of mesh (prosthetic vs biological) depends on the degree of contamination. Although prosthetic mesh offers the most durable repair, the risk of subsequent infection necessitating removal should be carefully considered, because mesh explantation is a morbid operation.

Under clean conditions in which a prosthetic is used, the next decision is whether to use a simple or composite mesh, and this is determined by whether the mesh comes into contact with bowel. Macroporous prosthetic is favored when there is no chance of contact, because the looser weave allows for superior host vascular ingrowth.

In cases of significant contamination, the safest choice for reinforcement is likely biological mesh.[58] However, in cases of bladder or bowel injury with minimal or no spillage, the risk of prosthetic infection may be sufficiently low to justify use of permanent synthetic material. One potential strategy is to place the patient on antibiotics and return to the operating room in several days for prosthetic mesh repair, assuming the absence of signs of infection, although this course of action has not been adequately studied. In cases of frank infection, it may be more cost-effective to consider an absorbable mesh rather than a biological graft, because the likelihood of recurrence is high no matter what type of mesh is used. In these cases of high-risk operations, postoperative wound complications are common (almost 50%) and should be anticipated.[47]

Once an appropriate mesh has been chosen, the final decision is the position of mesh placement: onlay, inlay (bridge), or underlay (intraperitoneal or retromuscular) (**Fig. 6**). Onlay mesh placement is favored by some because it avoids any chance of bowel contact and does not place any tension on the primary repair. However, it is generally discouraged because of the extensive subcutaneous dissection required and its attendant wound complications. In addition, the superficial location of the mesh theoretically increases the risk of mesh infection, and the recurrence rate is only marginally superior (if at all) to primary suture repair alone. Inlay mesh placement should be used only if primary tension-free fascial reapproximation is impossible despite CS, because this configuration is associated with high rates of recurrence.[46] It is our opinion (and that of the VHWG) that underlay mesh placement (retrorectus via the Rives-Stoppa technique) should be the default choice, because this method is associated with the lowest rate of wound complications and the lowest recurrence rate.[58,78,79] When affixing the mesh, it is important to ensure at least 4 cm of overlap on each side.[80] Recurrences rarely occur as a result of direct graft failure. The more common site of recurrence is laterally at the mesh-tissue interface.[81]

There have been several reports of the use of multilayered mesh repairs. For example, Petersen and colleagues[82] reported a series of 175 consecutive patients undergoing underlay prosthetic mesh repair of incisional hernias. In 50 cases, primary fascial reapproximation was not possible, and this group was further divided into

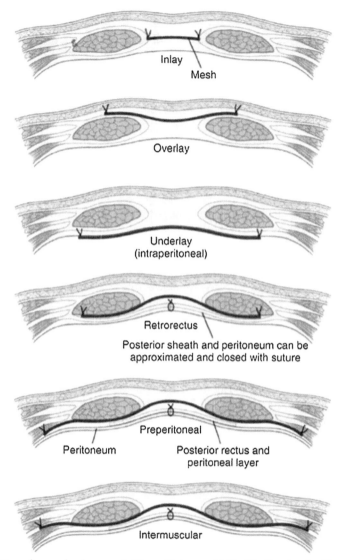

Fig. 6. Options for mesh placement. (*From* Malangoni MA, MJ. Hernias. In: Townsend RD, Beauchamp RD, Evers BM, et al, editors. Sabiston textbook of surgery: the biological basis of modern surgical practice. Philadelphia: Elsevier Saunders; 2012. p. 1133; with permission.)

those who had a second mesh placed as an inlay bridge and those without a mesh interposition. Although there was no significant difference in hernia recurrence rates, the investigators reported a significantly decreased mesh infection rate associated with the addition of the mesh interposition technique. A second technique, termed the pork sandwich, has been described, whereby porcine bioprosthesis is used in both underlay and overlay to reinforce a primary fascial closure after CS (**Fig. 7**). Satterwhite and colleagues[83] report using the pork sandwich on 19 patients, with no recurrences after a mean of 11 months, which compares favorably with a matched control group with 19% recurrence. Although these and other reports are interesting

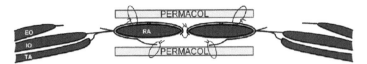

Fig. 7. Pork sandwich herniorrhaphy. (*From* Satterwhite TS, Miri S, Chung C, et al. Abdominal wall reconstruction with dual layer cross-linked porcine dermal xenograft: the "pork sandwich" herniorraphy. J Plast Reconstr Aesthet Surg 2012;65(3):333–41; with permission.)

and encouraging, the multilayered use of mesh has not been adequately studied to make recommendations for routine application.[84]

Parastomal hernias

A parastomal hernia is similar to other hernias of the anterior abdominal wall, with the added complicating factor of an intentional, permanent defect through the fascia and muscular layers. These hernias are common, and a 10-year longitudinal study reported that the parastomal herniation rate for ileostomies and colostomies is 16% and 36.7%, respectively, although most occur within the first 2 years.[85,86] It is generally agreed that stoma maturation through the rectus abdominis muscle, as opposed to lateral to the muscle, is associated with lower rates of herniation, although there is no high-quality evidence to support this belief.[87] However, aperture size has been shown to correlate with parastomal hernia, with a 10% increase in risk of hernia for every millimeter increase in stoma aperture size.[88] These hernias are well tolerated, and life-threatening complications are uncommon. Less than 20% of parastomal hernias require operative intervention, and, therefore, routine elective repair is not recommended. Parastomal contents are usually omentum, small bowel, or colon, although herniation of the gallbladder and stomach has been reported.[89,90] Indications for operation are local pain, poor appliance fit, severe prolapse, obstructive symptoms, incarceration, and rarely, cosmesis. More than half of parastomal hernia repairs are performed under emergent conditions.[91]

The same general principles apply: correct the life-threatening problem first, then attempt the safest and most durable hernia repair possible. Like all abdominal wall hernias, parastomal hernias can be repaired by several methods, including stoma relocation, and primary repair with or without mesh.

1. Stoma relocation: stoma relocation has been reported in the past as the optimal treatment. However, this exposes the patient to 3 potential sites of future herniation: the old stoma site, the new stoma site, and the laparotomy incision. With this approach, the recurrence rate at the stoma site is reported to be 33%. Incisional hernia at the accompanying laparotomy site occurs in more than 50%.[91]
2. Primary fascial repair: the advantage of this approach is that it does not require abdominal entry and should be reserved only for patients unable to tolerate laparotomy. This option is associated with predictably high recurrence rates (up to 76%) and is not generally recommended.[91,92]
3. Mesh reinforcement: first described by Sugarbaker in 1980, this option is associated with the lowest recurrence rate, especially with underlay mesh placement.[93,94] An additional consideration is whether to pass the stoma through the mesh via a keyhole incision or lateral to it (ie, the Sugarbaker technique) (**Fig. 8**).
   a. Prosthetic: despite concerns about mesh infection, studies have reported a surprisingly low rate of mesh-related complications (<5%) when used under elective conditions.[92] There have been occasional reports of mesh erosion into adjacent bowel.[95] Under emergent conditions, mesh selection should be

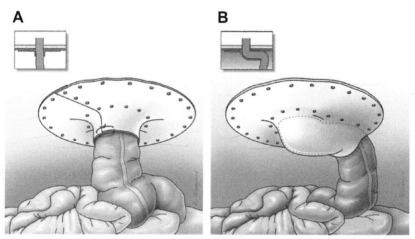

Fig. 8. (*A*) Keyhole technique for parastomal mesh placement. (*B*) Sugarbaker technique for parastomal mesh placement. (*From* Hansson BM, Slater NJ, van der Velden AS, et al. Surgical techniques for parastomal hernia repair: a systematic review of the literature. Ann Surg 2012;255(4):685–95; with permission.)

dictated by the degree of contamination. The prosthetic may be placed via a separate peritoneal incision, or directly, without laparotomy.[96–98]

b. Biological: there have been reports of use of porcine and human biological grafts to reinforce parastomal hernia repairs, but it is unclear how durable or cost-effective this approach is.[99,100]

Unusual hernias

Spigelian hernia Also known as spontaneous lateral VHs, hernia of the semilunar line, or hernias of the conjoint tendon, these hernias are rare, comprising approximately 1% of all abdominal wall hernias. They usually occur in the sixth or seventh decade of life, and both sexes are equally affected.[101] This eponymous hernia is named after the Belgian anatomist Adriaan van der Spiegal, who first described the semilunar line, where these hernias occur. Most (90%) spigelian hernias (SH) occur within the spigelian belt of Spangen, a transverse zone between the umbilicus and a line connecting the anterior superior iliac spines.[102]

The most common presenting symptom is localized pain, and diagnosis by physical examination is difficult, given the overlying external oblique muscle (ie, interparietal hernia). Point tenderness is often the only sign suggestive of the diagnosis. More than half are diagnosed intraoperatively. Ultrasonography or CT scan can help establish the diagnosis (**Fig. 9**). Because of the narrow neck, the risk of incarceration is high and it is recommended to electively repair all SH, because 20% to 30% require emergent operation.

The usual surgical approach is via a transverse incision directly overlying the hernia. Primary repair by suture repair of the internal oblique and transversus abdominis muscle may be accompanied with plug or mesh reinforcement.[103]

Lumbar hernias With less than 300 cases reported worldwide, spontaneous lumbar hernias are rare. Most hernias in this body region (80%) are acquired or incisional. Incarceration rarely occurs (<10%) because of the wide neck of the hernia orifice.[104–106] Both superior (Grynfeltt) lumbar triangle and inferior (Petit) lumbar triangle hernias show wide anatomic variation.[107,108] Operative repair is usually via an

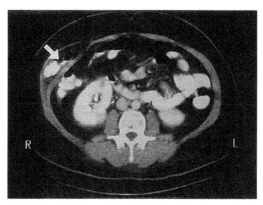

Fig. 9. Spigelian Hernia. (*From* Mukherjee K, Wise PE. Internal hernia through the gastrohepatic ligament after laparoscopic restorative proctocolectomy. Am Surg 2013;79(6):236–7.)

incision directly overlying the hernia. Although evidence is sparse, it is assumed that mesh repair is associated with lower recurrence rates than primary repair.

Obstructing diaphragmatic and internal hernia

Diaphragmatic hernia Diaphragmatic hernias (DH) occur through the diaphragm, the thin muscle separating the thoracic and abdominal cavities. Their natural history is to progressively enlarge over time, given the driving force of negative intra-thoracic pressure combined with positive intra-abdominal pressure. DH most commonly occur at the esophageal hiatus (hiatal DH), though congenital DH may occur elsewhere and traumatic DH may occur anywhere (**Fig. 10**).

DH may be classified as traumatic or nontraumatic. Nontraumatic hernias may be further subdivided as congenital or acquired. Congenital hernias are central, Bochdalek, and Morgagni. Central diaphragmatic defects (absence of the central tendon) are rare in adults and usually presents in infants.[109] Bochdalek hernias account for 90% of DH and occur through a defect in embryonic development. They occur more commonly on the left and have equal incidence in men and women. The most common presenting symptoms are pain and obstruction.[110] A foramen of Morgagni hernia is a

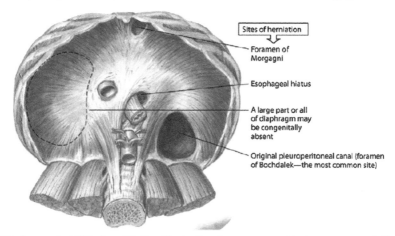

Fig. 10. Congenital DH sites. (Netter illustration from www.netterimages.com. © Elsevier Inc. All rights reserved.)

herniation through the space of Larrey, the area between the xiphoid process and the costal attachments of the diaphragm. Morgagni hernias account for <5% of nontraumatic DH in adults and the majority occur on the right side. The hernia sac most commonly contains omentum, transverse colon, or stomach.[111] Most are symptomatic and the condition affects women 3 times more commonly than men. Recurrence after repair is rare.[112]

Acquired DH are usually in the region of the esophageal hiatus.

Paraesophageal hernia The prototypical patient with paraesophageal hernia (PH) is frail and elderly, with significant comorbid medical illnesses, and perioperative morbidity and mortality are high, especially for emergent operations.[113] Untreated, approximately 30% of patients present with life-threatening complications.[114] There are 4 recognized types of PH, with type 1, or sliding hiatal hernia, predominating (>95%) **(Fig. 11)**. In type 2 and 3 PH, the fundus and potentially other parts of the stomach have herniated through the diaphragmatic hiatus, with a combined sliding hiatal hernia distinguishing type 3. A type 4 PH is defined as any PH that includes an additional intra-abdominal organ, such as spleen or colon.

Most patients report an antecedent history of symptoms, such as epigastric or substernal discomfort, dyspnea, nausea, or postprandial distress. Rarely, a patient may present with syncope or acute chest pain symptoms.[115] The estimated risk of requiring emergent operation for untreated PH is estimated at 1.16% per year, and a lifetime risk of 18% for patients older than 65 years.[116]

Obstructive symptoms, severe pulmonary dysfunction, and bleeding from ischemic or mechanical ulceration are the most common indications for emergent repair. The workup for a patient presenting with these symptoms is different from for a patient being considered for elective repair and generally includes plain films and CT of the chest and abdomen. Barium contrast studies, esophageal manometry, and 24-hour pH monitoring are not appropriate for acutely ill patients.

The steps for repair are identical for all DH: reduction of hernia contents, excision of hernia sac, and hernioplasty or herniorrhaphy (with or without mesh). For hiatal DH, additional considerations are whether to perform an antireflux procedure, or gastropexy. When performing surgery on the diaphragm, it is imperative to be aware of the course of the phrenic nerve and avoid division if possible. If primary repair is not possible, mesh selection is similar to VH repair: microporous prosthetic is preferred, followed by biological grafts in contaminated fields. Absorbable prosthetic mesh is never appropriate for DH repair. As with other external and internal hernias of the abdomen, the top priority is to correct the life-threatening problem; durable hiatal hernia repair is secondary. Because of the extensive vascular supply of the stomach,

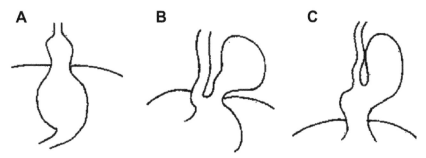

Fig. 11. Types of hiatal hernia. (*A*) Type 1, (*B*) Type 2, (*C*) Type 3. (*From* Oddsdottir M. Paraesophageal hernia. Surg Clin North Am 2000;80(4):1243–52; with permission.)

ischemia leading to necrosis is rare. The approach is usually transabdominal, although a transthoracic approach is advocated by some to permit additional esophageal mobilization and improve visualization during adhesiolysis. Rather than compromise exposure, the surgeon should not hesitate to perform a combined approach if necessary. The decision to attempt this operation laparoscopically should be determined on a case-by-case basis and should take into account the patient's physiologic status and experience of the surgeon. The peritoneal covering of the diaphragmatic crus should be preserved during dissection.

Once the hernia contents have been reduced and the hernia sac resected, attention is then directed toward repairing the diaphragmatic defect. Traditionally, this repair is accomplished via primary suture (nonabsorbable) reapproximation of the right and left diaphragmatic crura posterior to the esophagus, although 1 or 2 anterior sutures may be required in especially large defects. A tension-free repair is crucial. Autologous flap reinforcement with falciform ligament has been described (**Fig. 12**).[117]

Mesh reinforcement is recommended by some investigators, but robust evidence supporting its routine use is lacking. If it is considered, macroporous prosthetic should be avoided. Even with microporous prosthetics, erosion and stricture have been reported. The use of biological graft may be considered in certain cases, but this application is poorly studied.

The decision to perform an esophageal lengthening procedure, such as a Collis gastroplasty, should not be taken lightly, and every effort should be made to mobilize the esophagus transhiatally. Assuming that the gastroesophageal junction lies adequately below the hiatus, 1 final decision to consider is the addition of an antireflux procedure (such as a Nissen or Toupet fundoplication) or gastropexy to prevent recurrence.[118] Routine fundoplication in the absence of preoperative esophageal reflux symptoms is controversial.[119,120] Gastrostomy may be added as necessary for further intraperitoneal fixation of the stomach.

Internal hernia Internal hernias are rare, representing 2% of all hernias and less than 1% of all cases of bowel obstruction.[121] Delays in presentation, diagnosis, and treatment are common because of the vague nature of symptoms and difficulty in diagnosis. Overall mortality is estimated at 20%.[122] The 6 main types of internal

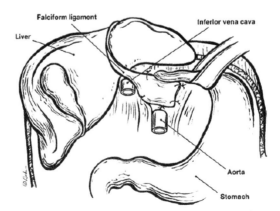

Fig. 12. Falciform ligament flap for crucal closure of hiatal hernia. (*From* Park AE, Hoogerboord CM, Sutton E. Use of the falciform ligament flap for closure of the esophageal hiatus in giant paraesophageal hernia. J Gastrointest Surg 2012;16(7):1417–21; with permission.)

abdominal hernias are, in order of decreasing frequency: paraduodenal, foramen of Winslow, transmesenteric, paracecal, intersigmoid, and paravesical (**Fig. 13**).[123]

Paraduodenal hernia Also known as Treitz hernia, paraduodenal hernia (PDH) accounts for more than 50% of internal hernias.[124] PDH are 3 times more common in men and occur most commonly on the left (75%), through the Landzert fossa.[124] The average age of presentation is between the third and fourth decades. The cause of PDH is unclear, but it is thought to be caused by either enlargement of a preexisting fossa or abnormal intestinal malrotation during embryonic development.

PDH most commonly presents as an acute bowel obstruction superimposed on a background of chronic, vague abdominal pain. Because of the rarity of the entity and the difficulty of diagnosis, a high level of suspicion must be maintained. It is estimated that the lifetime risk of bowel incarceration approaches 50%, and thus, these hernias should be repaired if discovered incidentally. Bowel necrosis occurs in 20% of emergent cases.[124]

Operative exploration may show the pathognomic empty abdomen sign, whereby only a segment of ileum is found in the peritoneal cavity, the remainder of the intestines being found within the hernia sac (**Fig. 14**). In right-sided PDH, the intestines herniate through the fossa of Waldeyer and are noted to lie posterior to the superior mesenteric artery (SMA).[125] For left-sided PDH, the border of the hernia sac contains the inferior mesenteric vein (IMV), and the anterior sac wall contains branches of the left colic artery.[126] As with all emergency hernia repairs, the first step is to reduce the intestine back into the peritoneal cavity, incising the constricting hernia ring if necessary, or opening the entire hernia sac. Because the hernia sac is formed by the mesocolon, in this case, the sac should be left in situ rather than excised. Extreme care should

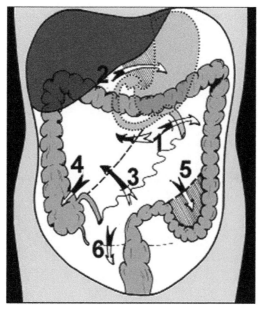

Fig. 13. Potential sites of internal herniation. 1, Paraduodenal; 2, Foramen of Winslow; 3, Transmesenteric; 4, Paracecal, 5, Para sigmoid; 6, Paravesical (pelvic). (*From* Ghahremani GG, Meyers MA. Internal abdominal hernias. Curr Probl Radiol 1975;5:1–30; with permission.)

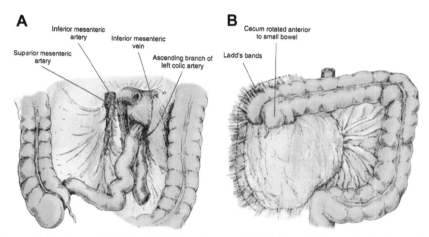

Fig. 14. (*A*) Left PDH. (*B*) Right PDH. (*From* Newsom BD, Kukora JS. Congenital and acquired internal hernias: unusual causes of small bowel obstruction. Am J Surg 1986;152(3):279–85; with permission.)

be taken to avoid injury to the IMV and SMA. The final step is to carefully close the hernia defect.

Foramen of Winslow hernia These hernias are rare, representing less than 10% of internal hernias.[127] Less than 200 cases have been reported worldwide (**Figs. 15** and **16**). The usual hernia contents are cecum and intestine, although a case of gallbladder herniation has been reported.[128] Because of delay in treatment, mortality can be as high as 49%.[129] The principles of treatment are identical to those for other internal hernias. Suture closure of the foramen is left to the discretion of the surgeon. There have been no reports of recurrence and injury to the portal triad structures is extremely morbid.

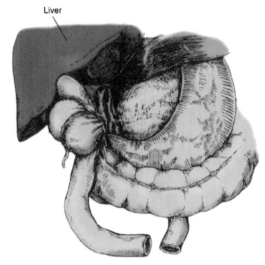

Fig. 15. Foramen of Winslow hernia. (*From* Newsom BD, Kukora JS. Congenital and acquired internal hernias: unusual causes of small bowel obstruction. Am J Surg 1986;152(3):279–85; with permission.)

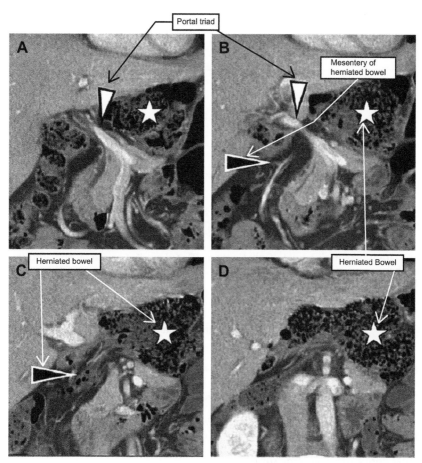

Fig. 16. (*A–D*), Sequential coronal images of Foramen of Winslow hernia. (*From* Azar AR, Abraham C, Coulier B, et al. Ileocecal herniation through the foramen of Winslow: MDCT diagnosis. Abdom Imaging 2010;35(5):574–7; with permission.)

Transmesenteric hernia Transmesenteric hernia (TMH) may be congenital or acquired, the former most commonly encountered in children.[130] They account for between 5% and 10% of internal hernias, and, in adults, are usually acquired after previous abdominal operations, trauma, or peritonitis. As in other internal hernias, palpable external defect is absent and the most common presenting symptoms are those suggestive of bowel obstruction. One interesting feature of TMH is that the bowel herniating through the mesenteric defect may exert such lateral pressure as to compress the vasculature in that mesentery, causing infarction of the unherniated bowel supplied by the mesentery (**Fig. 17**). Exploration is usually undertaken for a clinical condition, because CT scan is inaccurate in the preoperative diagnosis of TMH. The small bowel mesentery is usually involved, most commonly in the ileocecal region, although mesoappendiceal herniation has been reported.[127,131]

Paracecal hernia These hernias account for approximately 13% of internal hernias. A paracecal hernia is diagnosed preoperatively on CT by the presence of fluid-filled small intestine loops lateral to the cecum and posterior to the ascending colon

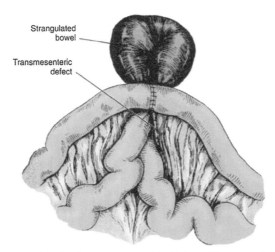

Fig. 17. Transmesenteric hernia. (*From* Newsom BD, Kukora JS. Congenital and acquired internal hernias: unusual causes of small bowel obstruction. Am J Surg 1986;152(3):279–85; with permission.)

(**Fig. 18**).[123,132] The principles of repair are similar to other internal and external hernias.

Intersigmoid hernia These hernias occur when intestines have herniated between adjacent segments of sigmoid colon and mesentery. The principles of repair are similar to other internal and external hernias.

Paravesical hernia These hernias are rare, with only about 60 cases reported worldwide. The principles of repair are similar to other internal and external hernias.[123]

Internal hernia after bariatric surgery

Special mention must be made of internal herniation after bariatric surgery, specifically Roux-en-Y gastric bypass, the most popular bariatric operation in the United

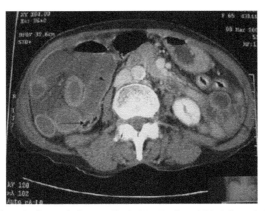

Fig. 18. Paracecal hernia (*arrow*). (*From* Choh NA, Rasheed M, Jehangir M. The computed tomography diagnosis of paracecal hernia. Hernia 2010;14(5):527–9; with permission.)

States. These internal hernias are the result of herniation through iatrogenic mesenteric defects and occur after 2.5% of bariatric operations. With increasing rates of weight-reduction operations being performed, the corresponding rates of internal hernia through mesenteric defects created as a result of gastrointestinal anastomosis have increased. Nonbariatric acute care surgeons may be called on to operate emergently on these patients, and a thorough understanding of the anatomy and potential sites of herniation is required (**Fig. 19**). These internal hernias most commonly present within the first postoperative month, but up to 25% can present after more than 1 year. Almost 90% occur within the first 2 years postoperatively.[133–136] Clinical diagnosis is difficult, with pain (usually upper quadrants) the most consistent symptom. Nausea and vomiting are frequent, but not universal. Diagnosis is usually made by CT scan or direct operative exploration. A mesenteric swirl has been reported as highly specific for internal herniation after gastric bypass.[137] Treatment consists of reduction, resection of necrotic intestine, and repair of the mesenteric defect with nonabsorbable suture to prevent future reherniation. Most are amenable to laparoscopic repair.[136,138]

Several technical factors have been found to increase the likelihood of postoperative internal herniation. Laparoscopic operations, compared with open operations, are associated with higher internal hernia rates, likely secondary to decreased adhesions, allowing for increased bowel mobility.[138,139] The retrocolic approach, by virtue of creation of an additional mesenteric defect, results in higher (up to 4-fold) internal herniation rates compared with antecolic.[134,135] Rapid postoperative excess weight loss has been associated with higher internal herniation risk.[133,135] The use of nonabsorbable suture for mesenteric closure at the index operation is associated with lower herniation rates compared with absorbable suture.[140]

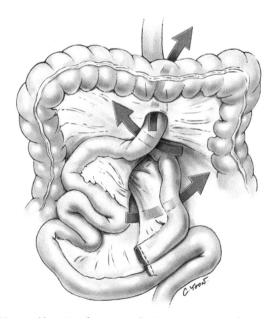

Fig. 19. Potential internal hernias after retrocolic Roux-en-Y gastric bypass. (*From* Carmody B, DeMaria E, Jamal M. Internal hernia after laparoscopic Roux-en-Y gastric bypass. Surg Obes Relat Dis 2005;1:543–8; with permission.)

Other internal hernias

Transomental hernia This rare entity involves herniation of small intestines through the gastrocolic greater omentum. An even rarer variant, the internal double omental hernia, involves further herniation of intestines through the gastrohepatic lesser omentum (**Fig. 20**). Intraoperatively, the omental defect is usually described as a constricting ring of stiff, fibrous tissue.[127] There is no hernia sac proper to limit the amount of bowel herniation, and this may account for the rapid develop of gangrene. The principles of repair are similar to other internal and external hernias.

Arcuate line hernia Although the presence of an ascending peritoneal fold between the posterior rectus sheath and the posterior aspect of the rectus abdominis muscle has been estimated to be present in up to 8% of the population, these internal hernias are rarely symptomatic, and only 7 cases have ever been reported (**Fig. 21**).[141,142] Misdiagnosis as the more lateral SH occurs in 50%.[143] Described repair techniques include incising the posterior rectus sheath to obliterate the internal hernia defect, and preperitoneal mesh repair.[144]

Broad ligament hernia This rare internal hernia in women has been reported less than 100 times in the world literature and is believed to result from trauma associated with previous pregnancy, because most occur in parous women.[145,146] After hernia reduction, treatment consists of either hernia defect repair or division of the fallopian tube and broad ligament.

Pelvic floor hernias

The 3 main pelvic floor hernias, in order of decreasing frequency, are: obturator, perineal, and sciatic.

Obturator hernia Obturator hernias (OH) are rare, representing less than 1% of abdominal wall hernias. They most commonly afflict thin, frail, elderly women.[147] Herniation of intestines through the obturator foramen of the bony pelvis presents a diagnostic challenge, because physical examination is highly insensitive because of the overlying pectineus muscle. Before the era of CT scanning, only 10% were diagnosed preoperatively. Occasionally, a palpable mass is evident on rectal or vaginal

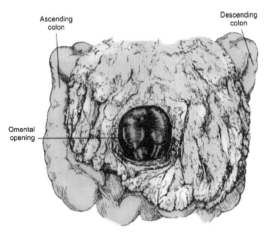

Fig. 20. Transomental hernia. (*From* Newsom BD, Kukora JS. Congenital and acquired internal hernias: unusual causes of small bowel obstruction. Am J Surg 1986;152(3):279–85; with permission.)

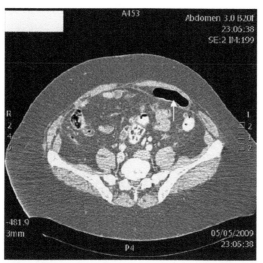

Fig. 21. Arcuate line hernia (*arrow*). (*From* Abasbassi M, Hendrickx T, Caluwé G, et al. Symptomatic linea arcuata hernia. Hernia 2011;15(2):229–31; with permission.)

examination. The pathognomonic Howship-Romberg sign (medial thigh pain on leg extension, adduction, or medial rotation) is specific for obturator nerve compression but is present in only one-third of patients.[147–149] The Hannington-Kiff sign (absence of the thigh adductor reflex) is more specific, but less well known and rarely tested.[150] In most patients (>90%), the presenting symptoms are abdominal pain and mechanical intestinal obstruction.[26] Because of delays in diagnosis, up to 75% of OH repairs require resection of infarcted bowel; morbidity and mortality are understandably high.[148] CT scan may show the lesion if the intestines are incarcerated (**Fig. 22**).[151]

Recently, a maneuver has been described to facilitate reduction of an incarcerated obturator hernia. With the patient lying supine, the leg is repeatedly flexed, externally rotated, and slightly adducted. Shigemitsu and colleagues[152] reported an 80% success rate with their technique, reducing an otherwise incarcerated OH and allowing for subsequent elective laparoscopic repair.

Although it is theoretically feasible to repair a known OH via an inguinal or thigh incision, full assessment of bowel viability may be limited, and therefore, laparotomy or laparoscopy is recommended. If the intestine cannot be reduced and the ring must be incised, care must be taken to avoid the obturator neurovascular bundle, which lies lateral to the sac in 50% of patients.[153] Primary repair may be difficult, because of the surrounding fixed bony structures, and a variety of repair techniques have been described, including plug,[154] prosthetic reinforcement, and autologous flap reinforcement.[155–157]

Perineal hernia Perineal hernia is a herniation through the pelvic diaphragm and is usually diagnosed in older, multiparous women. They may be repaired transabdominally, transperineally, or through a combined approach. Only approximately 100 cases have been reported in the literature. Repair is challenging, because of the complex anatomy of the pelvic floor, and may be accomplished via direct repair, autologous flap reconstruction, or mesh reinforcement.[158]

Sciatic hernia Sciatic hernia is defined as a herniation through the greater (suprapiriform or infrapiriform) or lesser sciatic foramen. Only about 100 cases have been

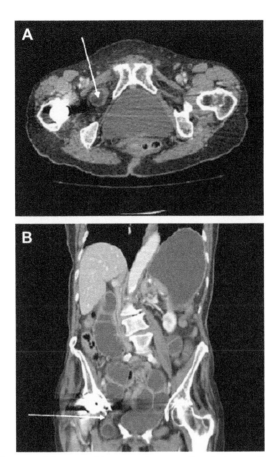

Fig. 22. (A) Axial image, (B) Coronal image. Obturator hernia (arrows). (From Galketiya K, Sakrepatna S, Gananadha S. Obturator hernia–an uncommon cause of small bowel obstruction. J Gastrointest Surg 2013;17(4):840–1; with permission.)

reported in the literature.[159] Most are acquired presumably secondary to increased intra-abdominal pressure. Presenting symptoms may include abdominal pain, a palpable buttock mass, or symptoms of sciatic nerve compression, and diagnosis is made via CT scan or operative exploration. Mesh repair (prosthetic or biological) is recommended.[160]

SUMMARY

Hernia emergencies are commonly encountered by the acute care surgeon. Although the location and contents may vary, the basic principles are constant: address the life-threatening problem first, then perform the safest and most durable hernia repair possible. Mesh reinforcement provides the most durable long-term results. Underlay positioning is associated with the best outcomes. CS is a useful technique to achieve tension-free primary fascial reapproximation. The choice of mesh is dictated by the degree of contamination. Internal herniation is rare, and preoperative diagnosis remains difficult. In all hernia emergencies, morbidity is high, and postoperative wound complications should be anticipated.

REFERENCES

1. Kingsnorth A, LeBlanc K. Hernias: inguinal and incisional. Lancet 2003; 362(9395):1561–71.
2. Dabbas N, Adams K, Pearson K, et al. Frequency of abdominal wall hernias: is classical teaching out of date? JRSM Short Rep 2011;2(1):5.
3. Kark AE, Kurzer M. Groin hernias in women. Hernia 2008;12(3):267–70.
4. Gallegos NC, Dawson J, Jarvis M, et al. Risk of strangulation in groin hernias. Br J Surg 1991;78(10):1171–3.
5. Fitzgibbons RJ, Giobbie-Hurder A, Gibbs JO. Watchful waiting vs. repair of inguinal hernia in minimally symptomatic men: a randomized clinical trial. JAMA 2006;295(3):285–92.
6. Fitzgibbons RJ Jr, Ramanan B, Arya S, et al. Long-term results of a randomized controlled trial of a nonoperative strategy (watchful waiting) for men with minimally symptomatic inguinal hernias. Ann Surg 2013;258:508–15.
7. Dahlstrand U, Wollert S, Nordin P, et al. Emergency femoral hernia repair: a study based on a national register. Ann Surg 2009;249(4):672–6.
8. Neumayer L, Giobbie-Hurder A, Jonasson O, et al. Open mesh versus laparoscopic mesh repair of inguinal hernia. N Engl J Med 2004;350(18):1819–27.
9. Hynes DM, Stroupe KT, Luo P, et al. Cost effectiveness of laparoscopic versus open mesh hernia operation: results of a Department of Veterans Affairs randomized clinical trial. J Am Coll Surg 2006;203(4):447–57.
10. Eklund AS, Montgomery AK, Rasmussen IC, et al. Low recurrence rate after laparoscopic (TEP) and open (Lichtenstein) inguinal hernia repair: a randomized, multicenter trial with 5-year follow-up. Ann Surg 2009;249(1):33–8.
11. Scott NW, McCormack K, Graham P, et al. Open mesh versus non-mesh for repair of femoral and inguinal hernia. Cochrane Database Syst Rev 2002;(4):CD002197.
12. Oida T, Kawasaki A, Mimatsu K, et al. Mesh vs. non-mesh repair for inguinal hernias in emergency operations. Hepatogastroenterology 2012;59(119):2112–4.
13. Nieuwenhuizen J, van Ramshorst GH, ten Brinke JG, et al. The use of mesh in acute hernia: frequency and outcome in 99 cases. Hernia 2011;15(3):297–300.
14. Rosen MJ, Krpata DM, Ermlich B, et al. A 5-year clinical experience with single-staged repairs of infected and contaminated abdominal wall defects utilizing biologic mesh. Ann Surg 2013;257(6):991–6.
15. Kouhia ST, Huttunen R, Silvasti SO, et al. Lichtenstein hernioplasty versus totally extraperitoneal laparoscopic hernioplasty in treatment of recurrent inguinal hernia–a prospective randomized trial. Ann Surg 2009;249(3):384–7.
16. Helgstrand F, Rosenberg J, Kehlet H, et al. Outcomes after emergency versus elective ventral hernia repair: a prospective nationwide study. World J Surg 2013;37(10):2273–9.
17. Muschaweck U. Umbilical and epigastric hernia repair. Surg Clin North Am 2003;83(5):1207–21.
18. Mudge MH, Hughes LE. Incisional hernia: a 10 year prospective study of incidence and attitude. Br J Surg 1985;72(1):70–1.
19. Bensley RP, Schermerhorn ML, Hurks R, et al. Risk of late-onset adhesions and incisional hernia repairs after surgery. J Am Coll Surg 2013;216(6):1159–67, 1167.e1–12.
20. Llaguna OH, Avgerinos DV, Lugo JZ, et al. Incidence and risk factors for the development of incisional hernia following elective laparoscopic versus open colon resections. Am J Surg 2010;200(2):265–9.

21. George CD, Ellis H. The results of incisional hernia repair: a twelve year review. Ann R Coll Surg Engl 1986;68(4):185–7.
22. Carlson MA, Ludwig KA, Condon RE. Ventral hernia and other complications of 1,000 midline incisions. South Med J 1995;88(4):450–3.
23. Read RC, Yoder G. Recent trends in the management of incisional herniation. Arch Surg 1989;124(4):485–8.
24. Derici H, Unalp HR, Bozdag AD, et al. Factors affecting morbidity and mortality in incarcerated abdominal wall hernias. Hernia 2007;11(4):341–6.
25. Nassar AH, Ashkar KA, Rashed AA, et al. Laparoscopic cholecystectomy and the umbilicus. Br J Surg 1997;84(5):630–3.
26. Salameh JR. Primary and unusual abdominal wall hernias. Surg Clin North Am 2008;88(1):45–60, viii.
27. Velasco M, Garcia-Ureña MA, Hidalgo M, et al. Current concepts on adult umbilical hernia. Hernia 1999;3:233–9.
28. Maniatis AG, Hunt CM. Therapy for spontaneous umbilical hernia rupture. Am J Gastroenterol 1995;90(2):310–2.
29. Chapman CS, Snell AM, Rowntree LG. Decompensated portal cirrhosis: report of one hundred and twelve cases. JAMA 1931;97(4):237–44.
30. O'Hara ET, Oliai A, Patek AJ Jr, et al. Management of umbilical hernias associated with hepatic cirrhosis and ascites. Ann Surg 1975;181(1):85–7.
31. Baron HC. Umbilical hernia secondary to cirrhosis of the liver. Complications of surgical correction. N Engl J Med 1960;263:824–8.
32. Pescovitz MD. Umbilical hernia repair in patients with cirrhosis. No evidence for increased incidence of variceal bleeding. Ann Surg 1984;199(3):325–7.
33. Gray SH, Vick CC, Graham LA, et al. Umbilical herniorrhapy in cirrhosis: improved outcomes with elective repair. J Gastrointest Surg 2008;12(4):675–81.
34. Choi SB, Hong KD, Lee JS, et al. Management of umbilical hernia complicated with liver cirrhosis: an advocate of early and elective herniorrhaphy. Dig Liver Dis 2011;43(12):991–5.
35. Choo EK, McElroy S. Spontaneous bowel evisceration in a patient with alcoholic cirrhosis and an umbilical hernia. J Emerg Med 2008;34(1):41–3.
36. Triantos CK, Kehagias I, Nikolopoulou V, et al. Incarcerated umbilical hernia after large volume paracentesis for refractory ascites. J Gastrointestin Liver Dis 2010;19(3):245.
37. Chu KM, McCaughan GW. Iatrogenic incarceration of umbilical hernia in cirrhotic patients with ascites. Am J Gastroenterol 1995;90(11):2058–9.
38. Lemmer JH, Strodel WE, Knol JA, et al. Management of spontaneous umbilical hernia disruption in the cirrhotic patient. Ann Surg 1983;198(1):30–4.
39. Runyon BA, Juler GL. Natural history of repaired umbilical hernias in patients with and without ascites. Am J Gastroenterol 1985;80(1):38–9.
40. O'Connor M, Allen JI, Schwartz ML. Peritoneovenous shunt therapy for leaking ascites in the cirrhotic patient. Ann Surg 1984;200(1):66–9.
41. Belghiti J, Durand F. Abdominal wall hernias in the setting of cirrhosis. Semin Liver Dis 1997;17(3):219–26.
42. Telem DA, Schiano T, Divino CM. Complicated hernia presentation in patients with advanced cirrhosis and refractory ascites: management and outcome. Surgery 2010;148(3):538–43.
43. Fagan SP, Awad SS, Berger DH. Management of complicated umbilical hernias in patients with end-stage liver disease and refractory ascites. Surgery 2004;135(6):679–82.

44. Slakey DP, Benz CC, Joshi S, et al. Umbilical hernia repair in cirrhotic patients: utility of temporary peritoneal dialysis catheter. Am Surg 2005;71(1):58–61.

45. Bachman S, Ramshaw B. Prosthetic material in ventral hernia repair: how do I choose? Surg Clin North Am 2008;88(1):101–12, ix.

46. Jin J, Rosen MJ, Blatnik J, et al. Use of acellular dermal matrix for complicated ventral hernia repair: does technique affect outcomes? J Am Coll Surg 2007;205(5):654–60.

47. Kim H, Bruen K, Vargo D. Acellular dermal matrix in the management of high-risk abdominal wall defects. Am J Surg 2006;192(6):705–9.

48. Patton JH Jr, Berry S, Kralovich KA. Use of human acellular dermal matrix in complex and contaminated abdominal wall reconstructions. Am J Surg 2007; 193(3):360–3 [discussion: 363].

49. Slater NJ, Hansson BM, Buyne OR, et al. Repair of parastomal hernias with biologic grafts: a systematic review. J Gastrointest Surg 2011;15(7):1252–8.

50. Shah BC, Tiwari MM, Goede MR, et al. Not all biologics are equal! Hernia 2011; 15(2):165–71.

51. de Castro Bras LE, Shurey S, Sibbons PD. Evaluation of crosslinked and noncrosslinked biologic prostheses for abdominal hernia repair. Hernia 2012; 16(1):77–89.

52. Primus FE, Harris HW. A critical review of biologic mesh use in ventral hernia repairs under contaminated conditions. Hernia 2013;17(1):21–30.

53. Ramirez OM, Ruas E, Dellon AL. "Components separation" method for closure of abdominal-wall defects: an anatomic and clinical study. Plast Reconstr Surg 1990;86(3):519–26.

54. de Vries Reilingh TS, van Goor H, Rosman C, et al. "Components separation technique" for the repair of large abdominal wall hernias. J Am Coll Surg 2003;196(1):32–7.

55. Yegiyants S, Tam M, Lee DJ, et al. Outcome of components separation for contaminated complex abdominal wall defects. Hernia 2012;16(1):41–5.

56. Morris LM, LeBlanc KA. Components separation technique utilizing an intraperitoneal biologic and an onlay lightweight polypropylene mesh: "a sandwich technique". Hernia 2013;17(1):45–51.

57. de Vries Reilingh TS, van Goor H, Charbon JA, et al. Repair of giant midline abdominal wall hernias: "components separation technique" versus prosthetic repair: interim analysis of a randomized controlled trial. World J Surg 2007; 31(4):756–63.

58. Breuing K, Butler CE, Ferzoco S, et al. Incisional ventral hernias: review of the literature and recommendations regarding the grading and technique of repair. Surgery 2010;148(3):544–58.

59. Espinosa-de-los-Monteros A, Dominguez I, Zamora-Valdes D, et al. Closure of midline contaminated and recurrent incisional hernias with components separation technique reinforced with plication of the rectus muscles. Hernia 2013;17(1):75–9.

60. Rosen MJ, Jin J, McGee MF, et al. Laparoscopic component separation in the single-stage treatment of infected abdominal wall prosthetic removal. Hernia 2007;11(5):435–40.

61. Giurgius M, Bendure L, Davenport DL, et al. The endoscopic component separation technique for hernia repair results in reduced morbidity compared to the open component separation technique. Hernia 2012;16(1):47–51.

62. Lowe JB, Garza JR, Bowman JL, et al. Endoscopically assisted "components separation" for closure of abdominal wall defects. Plast Reconstr Surg 2000; 105(2):720–9 [quiz: 730].

63. Milburn ML, Shah PK, Friedman EB, et al. Laparoscopically assisted components separation technique for ventral incisional hernia repair. Hernia 2007; 11(2):157–61.

64. Krpata DM, Blatnik JA, Novitsky YW, et al. Posterior and open anterior components separations: a comparative analysis. Am J Surg 2012;203(3):318–22.

65. van Geffen HJ, Simmermacher RK, Bosscha K, et al. Anatomical considerations for surgery of the anterolateral abdominal wall. Hernia 2004;8(2):93–7.

66. Carbonell AM, Cobb WS, Chen SM. Posterior components separation during retromuscular hernia repair. Hernia 2008;12(4):359–62.

67. Mayo WJ. VI. An operation for the radical cure of umbilical hernia. Ann Surg 1901;34(2):276–80.

68. Luijendijk RW, Lemmen MH, Hop WC, et al. Incisional hernia recurrence following "vest-over-pants" or vertical Mayo repair of primary hernias of the midline. World J Surg 1997;21(1):62–5 [discussion: 66].

69. Paul A, Korenkov M, Peters S, et al. Unacceptable results of the Mayo procedure for repair of abdominal incisional hernias. Eur J Surg 1998;164(5):361–7.

70. Arroyo A, Garcia P, Perez F, et al. Randomized clinical trial comparing suture and mesh repair of umbilical hernia in adults. Br J Surg 2001;88(10):1321–3.

71. Ammar SA. Management of complicated umbilical hernias in cirrhotic patients using permanent mesh: randomized clinical trial. Hernia 2010;14(1):35–8.

72. Perrakis E, Velimezis G, Vezakis A, et al. A new tension-free technique for the repair of umbilical hernia, using the Prolene hernia system–early results from 48 cases. Hernia 2003;7(4):178–80.

73. Khera G, Berstock DA. Incisional, epigastric and umbilical hernia repair using the Prolene hernia system: describing a novel technique. Hernia 2006;10(4): 367–9.

74. Luijendijk RW, Hop WC, van den Tol MP, et al. A comparison of suture repair with mesh repair for incisional hernia. N Engl J Med 2000;343(6):392–8.

75. Burger JW, Luijendijk RW, Hop WC, et al. Long-term follow-up of a randomized controlled trial of suture versus mesh repair of incisional hernia. Ann Surg 2004; 240(4):578–83 [discussion: 583–5].

76. Sauerland S, Schmedt CG, Lein S, et al. Primary incisional hernia repair with or without polypropylene mesh: a report on 384 patients with 5-year follow-up. Langenbecks Arch Surg 2005;390(5):408–12.

77. Voeller GR, Ramshaw B, Park AE, et al. Incisional hernia. J Am Coll Surg 1999; 189(6):635–7.

78. Duce AM, Mugüerza JM, Villeta R, et al. The Rives operation for the repair of incisional hernias. Hernia 1997;1:175–7.

79. Stoppa RE. The treatment of complicated groin and incisional hernias. World J Surg 1989;13(5):545–54.

80. Binnebosel M, Rosch R, Junge K, et al. Biomechanical analyses of overlap and mesh dislocation in an incisional hernia model in vitro. Surgery 2007;142(3): 365–71.

81. Shell DH, de la Torre J, Andrades P, et al. Open repair of ventral incisional hernias. Surg Clin North Am 2008;88(1):61–83, viii.

82. Petersen S, Henke G, Zimmermann L, et al. Ventral rectus fascia closure on top of mesh hernia repair in the sublay technique. Plast Reconstr Surg 2004;114(7): 1754–60.

83. Satterwhite TS, Miri S, Chung C, et al. Abdominal wall reconstruction with dual layer cross-linked porcine dermal xenograft: the "pork sandwich" herniorraphy. J Plast Reconstr Aesthet Surg 2012;65(3):333–41.

84. Kolker AR, Brown DJ, Redstone JS, et al. Multilayer reconstruction of abdominal wall defects with acellular dermal allograft (AlloDerm) and component separation. Ann Plast Surg 2005;55(1):36–41 [discussion: 41–2].
85. Londono-Schimmer EE, Leong AP, Phillips RK. Life table analysis of stomal complications following colostomy. Dis Colon Rectum 1994;37(9):916–20.
86. Leong AP, Londono-Schimmer EE, Phillips RK. Life-table analysis of stomal complications following ileostomy. Br J Surg 1994;81(5):727–9.
87. Sjodahl R, Anderberg B, Bolin T. Parastomal hernia in relation to site of the abdominal stoma. Br J Surg 1988;75(4):339–41.
88. Pilgrim CH, McIntyre R, Bailey M. Prospective audit of parastomal hernia: prevalence and associated comorbidities. Dis Colon Rectum 2010;53(1):71–6.
89. Garcia RM, Brody F, Miller J, et al. Parastomal herniation of the gallbladder. Hernia 2005;9(4):397–9.
90. Carne PW, Robertson GM, Frizelle FA. Parastomal hernia. Br J Surg 2003;90(7): 784–93.
91. Rubin MS, Schoetz DJ Jr, Matthews JB. Parastomal hernia. Is stoma relocation superior to fascial repair? Arch Surg 1994;129(4):413–8 [discussion: 418–9].
92. Hansson BM, Slater NJ, van der Velden AS, et al. Surgical techniques for parastomal hernia repair: a systematic review of the literature. Ann Surg 2012;255(4): 685–95.
93. Sugarbaker PH. Prosthetic mesh repair of large hernias at the site of colonic stomas. Surg Gynecol Obstet 1980;150(4):576–8.
94. Janes A, Cengiz Y, Israelsson LA. Preventing parastomal hernia with a prosthetic mesh: a 5-year follow-up of a randomized study. World J Surg 2009; 33(1):118–21 [discussion: 122–3].
95. Aldridge AJ, Simson JN. Erosion and perforation of colon by synthetic mesh in a recurrent paracolostomy hernia. Hernia 2001;5(2):110–2.
96. Sugarbaker PH. Peritoneal approach to prosthetic mesh repair of paraostomy hernias. Ann Surg 1985;201(3):344–6.
97. Meyer C, de Manzini N, Rohr S, et al. A direct approach for the treatment of parastomal hernias using a prosthesis. A report of 15 cases. Hernia 1997;1:89–92.
98. Martinez-Munive A, Medina-Ramirez Llaca O, Quijano-Orvananos F, et al. Intraparietal mesh repair for parastomal hernias. Hernia 2000;4:272–4.
99. Smart NJ, Velineni R, Khan D, et al. Parastomal hernia repair outcomes in relation to stoma site with diisocyanate cross-linked acellular porcine dermal collagen mesh. Hernia 2011;15(4):433–7.
100. Taner T, Cima RR, Larson DW, et al. The use of human acellular dermal matrix for parastomal hernia repair in patients with inflammatory bowel disease: a novel technique to repair fascial defects. Dis Colon Rectum 2009;52(2):349–54.
101. Montes IS, Deysine M. Spigelian and other uncommon hernia repairs. Surg Clin North Am 2003;83(5):1235–53, viii.
102. Spangen L. Spigelian hernia. World J Surg 1989;13(5):573–80.
103. Tsalis K, Zacharakis E, Lambrou I, et al. Incarcerated small bowel in a spigelian hernia. Hernia 2004;8(4):384–6.
104. Teo KA, Burns E, Garcea G, et al. Incarcerated small bowel within a spontaneous lumbar hernia. Hernia 2010;14(5):539–41.
105. Moreno-Egea A, Baena EG, Calle MC, et al. Controversies in the current management of lumbar hernias. Arch Surg 2007;142(1):82–8.
106. Astarcioglu H, Sokmen S, Atila K, et al. Incarcerated inferior lumbar (Petit's) hernia. Hernia 2003;7(3):158–60.

107. Loukas M, El-Zammar D, Shoja MM, et al. The clinical anatomy of the triangle of Grynfeltt. Hernia 2008;12(3):227–31.
108. Loukas M, Tubbs RS, El-Sedfy A, et al. The clinical anatomy of the triangle of Petit. Hernia 2007;11(5):441–4.
109. Jagad RB, Kamani P. Central diaphragmatic hernia in an adult: a rare presentation. Hernia 2012;16(5):607–9.
110. Brown SR, Horton JD, Trivette E, et al. Bochdalek hernia in the adult: demographics, presentation, and surgical management. Hernia 2011;15(1):23–30.
111. Altinkaya N, Parlakgumus A, Koc Z, et al. Morgagni hernia: diagnosis with multidetector computed tomography and treatment. Hernia 2010;14(3): 277–81.
112. Iso Y, Sawada T, Rokkaku K, et al. A case of symptomatic Morgagni's hernia and a review of Morgagni's hernia in Japan (263 reported cases). Hernia 2006;10(6): 521–4.
113. Poulose BK, Gosen C, Marks JM, et al. Inpatient mortality analysis of paraesophageal hernia repair in octogenarians. J Gastrointest Surg 2008;12(11): 1888–92.
114. Oddsdottir M. Paraesophageal hernia. Surg Clin North Am 2000;80(4):1243–52.
115. Maekawa T, Suematsu M, Shimada T, et al. Unusual swallow syncope caused by huge hiatal hernia. Intern Med 2002;41(3):199–201.
116. Stylopoulos N, Gazelle GS, Rattner DW. Paraesophageal hernias: operation or observation? Ann Surg 2002;236(4):492–500 [discussion: 500–1].
117. Park AE, Hoogerboord CM, Sutton E. Use of the falciform ligament flap for closure of the esophageal hiatus in giant paraesophageal hernia. J Gastrointest Surg 2012;16(7):1417–21.
118. Fuller CB, Hagen JA, DeMeester TR, et al. The role of fundoplication in the treatment of type II paraesophageal hernia. J Thorac Cardiovasc Surg 1996;111(3): 655–61.
119. Rakic S, Pesko P, Dunjic MS, et al. Paraoesophageal hernia repair with and without concomitant fundoplication. Br J Surg 1994;81(8):1162–3.
120. Williamson WA, Ellis FH Jr, Streitz JM Jr, et al. Paraesophageal hiatal hernia: is an antireflux procedure necessary? Ann Thorac Surg 1993;56(3):447–51 [discussion: 451–2].
121. Martin LC, Merkle EM, Thompson WM. Review of internal hernias: radiographic and clinical findings. AJR Am J Roentgenol 2006;186(3):703–17.
122. Fan HP, Yang AD, Chang YJ, et al. Clinical spectrum of internal hernia: a surgical emergency. Surg Today 2008;38(10):899–904.
123. Mathieu D, Luciani A. Internal abdominal herniations. AJR Am J Roentgenol 2004;183(2):397–404.
124. Zonca P, Maly T, Mole DJ, et al. Treitz's hernia. Hernia 2008;12(5):531–4.
125. Hong SS, Kim AY, Kim PN, et al. Current diagnostic role of CT in evaluating internal hernia. J Comput Assist Tomogr 2005;29(5):604–9.
126. Davis R. Surgery of left paraduodenal hernia. Am J Surg 1975;129(5):570–3.
127. Newsom BD, Kukora JS. Congenital and acquired internal hernias: unusual causes of small bowel obstruction. Am J Surg 1986;152(3):279–85.
128. Dardik H, Cowen R. Herniation of the gallbladder through the epiploic foramen into the lesser sac. Ann Surg 1967;165(4):644–6.
129. Osvaldt AB, Mossmann DF, Bersch VP, et al. Intestinal obstruction caused by a foramen of Winslow hernia. Am J Surg 2008;196(2):242–4.
130. Gomes R, Rodrigues J. Spontaneous adult transmesentric hernia with bowel gangrene. Hernia 2011;15(3):343–5.

131. Rooney JA, Carroll JP, Keeley JL. Internal hernias due to defects in the meso-appendix and mesentery of small bowel, and probable Ivemark syndrome: report of two cases. Ann Surg 1963;157(2):254–8.

132. Choh NA, Rasheed M, Jehangir M. The computed tomography diagnosis of par-acecal hernia. Hernia 2010;14(5):527–9.

133. Schneider C, Cobb W, Scott J, et al. Rapid excess weight loss following laparo-scopic gastric bypass leads to increased risk of internal hernia. Surg Endosc 2011;25(5):1594–8.

134. Champion JK, Williams M. Small bowel obstruction and internal hernias after laparoscopic Roux-en-Y gastric bypass. Obes Surg 2003;13(4):596–600.

135. Ahmed AR, Rickards G, Husain S, et al. Trends in internal hernia incidence after laparoscopic Roux-en-Y gastric bypass. Obes Surg 2007;17(12):1563–6.

136. Garza E Jr, Kuhn J, Arnold D, et al. Internal hernias after laparoscopic Roux-en-Y gastric bypass. Am J Surg 2004;188(6):796–800.

137. Lockhart ME, Tessler FN, Canon CL, et al. Internal hernia after gastric bypass: sensitivity and specificity of seven CT signs with surgical correlation and con-trols. AJR Am J Roentgenol 2007;188(3):745–50.

138. Iannelli A, Facchiano E, Gugenheim J. Internal hernia after laparoscopic Roux-en-Y gastric bypass for morbid obesity. Obes Surg 2006;16:1265–71.

139. Higa KD, Ho T, Boone KB. Internal hernias after laparoscopic Roux-en-Y gastric bypass: incidence, treatment and prevention. Obes Surg 2003;13(3):350–4.

140. Paroz A, Calmes JM, Giusti V, et al. Internal hernia after laparoscopic Roux-en-Y gastric bypass for morbid obesity: a continuous challenge in bariatric surgery. Obes Surg 2006;16(11):1482–7.

141. Montgomery A, Petersson U, Austrums E. The arcuate line hernia: operative treatment and a review of the literature. Hernia 2013;17(3):391–6.

142. Coulier B. Multidetector computed tomography features of linea arcuata (arcuate-line of Douglas) and linea arcuata hernias. Surg Radiol Anat 2007; 29(5):397–403.

143. von Meyenfeldt EM, van Keulen EM, Eerenberg JP, et al. The linea arcuata her-nia: a report of two cases. Hernia 2010;14(2):207–9.

144. Abasbassi M, Hendrickx T, Caluwe G, et al. Symptomatic linea arcuata hernia. Hernia 2011;15(2):229–31.

145. Chapman VM, Rhea JT, Novelline RA. Internal hernia through a defect in the broad ligament: a rare cause of intestinal obstruction. Emerg Radiol 2003; 10(2):94–5.

146. Langan RC, Holzman K, Coblentz M. Strangulated hernia through a defect in the broad ligament: a sheep in wolf's clothing. Hernia 2012;16(4):481–3.

147. Nasir BS, Zendejas B, Ali SM, et al. Obturator hernia: the Mayo Clinic experi-ence. Hernia 2012;16(3):315–9.

148. Rodriguez-Hermosa JI, Codina-Cazador A, Maroto-Genover A, et al. Obturator hernia: clinical analysis of 16 cases and algorithm for its diagnosis and treat-ment. Hernia 2008;12(3):289–97.

149. Skandalakis LJ, Skandalakis PN, Colborn GL, et al. Obturator hernia: embry-ology, anatomy, surgery. Hernia 2000;4:121–8.

150. Hannington-Kiff JG. Absent thigh adductor reflex in obturator hernia. Lancet 1980;1(8161):180.

151. Galketiya K, Sakrepatna S, Gananadha S. Obturator hernia–an uncommon cause of small bowel obstruction. J Gastrointest Surg 2013;17(4):840–1.

152. Shigemitsu Y, Akagi T, Morimoto A, et al. The maneuver to release an incarcer-ated obturator hernia. Hernia 2012;16(6):715–7.

153. Skandalakis LJ, Androulakis J, Colborn GL, et al. Obturator hernia. Embryology, anatomy, and surgical applications. Surg Clin North Am 2000;80(1):71–84.
154. Martinez Insua C, Costa Pereira JM, Cardoso de Oliveira M. Obturator hernia: the plug technique. Hernia 2001;6:161–3.
155. Tchanque CN, Virmani S, Teklehaimanot N, et al. Bilateral obturator hernia with intestinal obstruction: repair with a cigar roll technique. Hernia 2010;14(5): 543–5.
156. Maharaj D, Maharaj S, Young L, et al. Obturator hernia repair–a new technique. Hernia 2002;6(1):45–7.
157. Shipkov CD, Uchikov AP, Grigoriadis E. The obturator hernia: difficult to diagnose, easy to repair. Hernia 2004;8(2):155–7.
158. Preiss A, Herbig B, Dorner A. Primary perineal hernia: a case report and review of the literature. Hernia 2006;10(5):430–3.
159. Losanoff JE, Basson MD, Gruber SA, et al. Sciatic hernia: a comprehensive review of the world literature (1900-2008). Am J Surg 2010;199(1):52–9.
160. Chaudhuri A, Chye KK, Marsh SK. Sciatic hernias: choice of optimal prosthetic repair material in preventing long-term morbidity. Hernia 1999;4:229–31.

Management of the Open Abdomen

Demetrios Demetriades, MD, PhD[a],*, Ali Salim, MD[b]

KEYWORDS

- Damage control • Intra-abdominal hypertension • Peritoneal sepsis
- Open abdomen • Temporary abdominal closure • Enteroatmospheric fistula

KEY POINTS

- Routine monitoring of bladder pressures in high-risk patients should be a standard intensive care unit (ICU) protocol.
- Intra-abdominal hypertension (IAH) produces toxic lymph, which causes organ dysfunction. Early release of the IAH and effective removal of the toxic lymph improve outcomes.
- Damage control should be considered early, before the patient reaches the extremis stage.
- Although the open abdomen is a strong weapon in the surgeon's armamentarium, it is also associated with serious complications, such as severe fluid and protein loss, nutritional problems, enteroatmospheric fistulas, and development of massive incisional hernias. The most effective way to prevent or reduce these complications is to close the abdominal wall as soon as possible.
- In severe abdominal sepsis, the open abdomen, using traditional abdominal packing, is of no benefit and might be associated with increased mortality and a higher incidence of enteroatmospheric fistulas. However, there is evidence that negative pressure therapy in these cases improves outcomes.
- Numerous techniques may be used for temporary abdominal closure. They include the Bogota bag, the Wittmann patch, absorbable synthetic meshes, and various negative pressure therapy techniques. Each technique has its own advantages and disadvantages.
- The development of an enteroatmospheric fistula increases the ICU stay by 3-fold, the hospital stay by 4-fold, and the hospital charges by 4.5-fold. The most effective way to prevent this complication is early closure of the abdominal wall. The management strategy should include temporary local control to prevent spillage of enteric contents on the surrounding tissues, while planning the definitive closure of the fistula.

[a] Division of Acute Care Surgery, Department of Surgery, University of Southern California, Los Angeles, CA, USA; [b] Division of Trauma, Burns, and Surgical Critical Care, Brigham and Women's Hospital, Boston, MA, USA
* Corresponding author.
E-mail address: demetria@usc.edu

Surg Clin N Am 94 (2014) 131–153
http://dx.doi.org/10.1016/j.suc.2013.10.010
0039-6109/14/$ – see front matter © 2014 Elsevier Inc. All rights reserved.

INTRODUCTION

The management of complex abdominal problems with the open-abdomen and temporary abdominal closure techniques has become a common and valuable tool in surgery. Damage control for life-threatening intra-abdominal bleeding, early recognition and treatment of intra-abdominal hypertension (IAH) and abdominal compartment syndrome (ACS), and new strategies in the management of severe intra-abdominal sepsis have resulted in a major increase in the number of cases treated with an open abdomen. Although the open abdomen is usually effective in addressing the primary disorder, it is also associated with serious complications, such as severe fluid and protein loss, nutritional problems, enteroatmospheric fistulas, fascial retraction with loss of abdominal domain, and development of massive incisional hernias (**Box 1**). The initial management of the open abdomen may determine the frequency, severity, and duration of these complications and have a significant effect on survival.

Indications for the Open Abdomen

There are 3 major indications for the use of the open-abdomen technique: (1) prevention or treatment of the ACS, (2) damage control for life-threatening intra-abdominal bleeding, and (3) management of severe intra-abdominal sepsis.

IAH and ACS

IAH and ACS are commonly encountered among both surgical and nonsurgical critically ill patients. Although IAH is defined as a sustained pathologic increase in intra-abdominal pressure (IAP) greater than or equal to 12 mm Hg, ACS is defined as a sustained increase in IAP greater than 20 mm Hg that is associated with new organ dysfunction/failure. Analogous to cerebral perfusion pressure, abdominal perfusion pressure (APP; mean arterial pressure [MAP] – IAP) is a measure of the net pressure available for perfusion of intra-abdominal organs. A target APP associated with appropriate perfusion is 60 mm Hg.

Classification

IAP is defined as the steady-state pressure concealed within the abdominal wall. For most critically ill patients, an IAP of 5 to 7 mm Hg is considered normal. Although the exact pressure that defines IAH is debated, most studies show a decrease in visceral organ perfusion at an IAP of 10 to 15 mm Hg. Thus, if left untreated, prolonged increases in IAP could result in multisystem organ failure.

In defining the severity of IAP, the World Congress on Abdominal Compartment Syndrome introduced a useful grading system for IAH: grade I (IAP 12–15 mm Hg), grade II (IAP 16–20 mm Hg), grade III (IAP 21–25 mm Hg), and grade IV (IAP>25 mm

---

Box 1
Problems associated with the open abdomen

- Fluid and protein loss
- Malnutrition
- Enteroatmospheric fistulas
- Loss of abdominal wall domain
- Prolonged intensive care unit and hospital stay
- Increased hospital costs

Hg). In contrast with IAH, ACS is not graded; however, it is classified as primary, secondary, or recurrent ACS.

Primary ACS is most commonly encountered and occurs from a primary intra-abdominal cause such as abdominal trauma, pancreatitis, mesenteric venous obstruction, ascites, retroperitoneal hemorrhage, or ruptured abdominal aortic aneurysm. Secondary ACS or extra-abdominal syndrome refers to ACS that results from massive bowel edema from sepsis, capillary leak, massive fluid resuscitation, or burns. Recurrent ACS occurs after resolution of primary or secondary ACS and usually results from abdominal closure in an edematous patient with an open abdomen.

Prevalence and epidemiology
The prevalence of ACS varies among populations. In 2002, Hong and colleagues prospectively evaluated 706 patients admitted to a trauma intensive care unit (ICU) over a 9-month period and found IAH and ACS among 2% and 1% of the patients, respectively. In patients with severe abdominal or pelvic trauma who had undergone a damage-control laparotomy with subsequent primary fascial closure, the incidence of ACS increased to 5.5%. Although most frequently studied in the context of trauma, Malbrain and colleagues studied the prevalence of ACS in 97 patients at 13 different medical, surgical, and 24 trauma units over 6 different counties. Fifty-eight percent of the patients had an IAH of 12 mm Hg or greater, 30% had severe IAH of 15 mm Hg or more, and 8% of patients had ACS with IAH more than 20 mm Hg with organ failure. The mortality is high, ranging from 60% to 70%, caused by the presence of multiorgan failure and severe underlying injuries.

There is evidence that changes in resuscitation introduced in the past few years have decreased the incidence and mortality of ACS. These changes include a more balanced transfusion protocol (including 1:1 ratios), limited use of crystalloid resuscitation, and widespread use of damage-control approaches.

Pathophysiology
The molecular and cellular events that lead to ACS are multifactorial. As described by Walker and Criddle, blood is shunted away from the gastrointestinal tract toward the heart and brain in shock states. This shunting of blood leads to cellular hypoxia within the tissues of the intestine. This cellular hypoxia results in the release of proinflammatory cytokines that promote vasodilation and increased capillary permeability, leading to edema. After cellular reperfusion, oxygen free radicals are generated, which results in insufficient oxygen delivery to the tissues, thus limiting the production of adenosine triphosphate and impairing energy-dependent cellular activity. The sodium-potassium pump fails, and sodium leaks into the cells drawing water into the cell. The cell swells, the membrane loses its integrity, and intracellular contents are then spilled into extracellular space causing inflammation, increased capillary permeability, and edema. IAP quickly increases and intestinal perfusion is impaired.

IAH affects multiple organ systems. Increase in IAP results in an increase in thoracic pressure and diaphragmatic elevation, causing a reduction in chest wall compliance, total lung capacity, and functional residual volume, which leads to hypoxia, hypercapnia, and the need for mechanical ventilation with increased intrathoracic pressure. Increased IAP also directly compresses the inferior vena cava and portal vein, leading to an increase in systemic afterload, decreased hepatosplanchnic flow with impaired liver function, decreased stroke volume, and a reduction in cardiac output. A reduction in cardiac output results in renal insufficiency secondary to prerenal azotemia, as well as intestinal ischemia and infarction caused by a decrease in mesenteric and intestinal mucosal blood flow. Renal parenchymal compression with its resultant compression of renal arterioles and veins increases renal vascular resistance and diminishes renal blood flow. This reduction of renal blood flow and glomerular filtration from the combination of prerenal and renal changes results in alterations of circulating renin, antidiuretic hormone, and aldosterone, further altering renal and systemic vascular resistance. In addition to a reduction in cardiac output, there is an impairment of lymphatic flow and a subsequent increase in intestinal edema.

Clinical manifestations of ACS include a distended and tense abdomen associated with increased airway pressures with progressive hypoxia and hypercapnia, increased heart rate with hypotension, and impaired renal function with oliguria that progresses to anuria without appropriate therapy. Increased intracranial pressure has also been described, probably caused by an increased intrathoracic pressure resulting in a functional obstruction to cerebral venous outflow.

Risk factors
Risk factors are in 4 distinct categories: diminished abdominal wall compliance, increased intraluminal contents, increased abdominal contents, and capillary leak/fluid resuscitation. Independent risk factors for primary ACS include the administration of more than 5 L of crystalloid infusion within 24 hours, the transfusion of more than 10 units of packed red blood cell transfusions in a 24-hour period, hypothermia (<33°C), acidosis (base deficit < -14 mmol/L; pH <7.2), and body mass index (>30). For patients with burns, greater than 30% of the total body surface area (TBSA) burn is a risk factor for IAH, whereas greater than 50% TBSA and inhalation injury are risk factors for ACS.

Diagnosis
A high index of suspicion is necessary to make the diagnosis in a timely fashion, preferably before IAH progresses to ACS. According to the World Society of the Abdominal Compartment Syndrome 2013 consensus guidelines, IAP should be measured when there are greater than or equal to 2 known risk factor for IAH/ACS in critically ill or injured patients. After a baseline measurement, serial measurements are then performed during the patient's critical illness. Although a variety of methods to measure the IAP have been described, measuring the bladder pressure is considered the gold standard. The intravesicular instillation volume should be a maximum of 25 mL saline (in children, 1 mL/kg, maximum 25 mL) to avoid overdistention and falsely increased IAP. The IAP should then be measured at end-expiration with the patient supine and the transducer zeroed at the midaxillary line. Although the critical IAP that defines ACS is debatable, ACS is present with a sustained IAP greater than 20 mm Hg associated with any new organ dysfunction or failure.

Management and treatment
Four principles for the management of IAP are advised: serial monitoring of IAP, optimization of systemic perfusion and organ function in the patient with increased IAP, institution of specific medical procedures to reduce IAP, and prompt surgical decompressive laparotomy for refractory IAH.

Sedation, analgesia, and neuromuscular blockade can be used to decrease IAP. Early goal-directed fluid resuscitation is critical to correct hypovolemia and thus prevent end-organ failure. However, careful attention to avoiding a positive fluid balance is warranted given the risk of the detrimental effects of worsening IAP with increased fluids. Drainage of any significant ascites, a common problem in extensive burns, may reduce the IAP. Abdominal decompression via decompressive laparotomy is the standard treatment of refractory IAH and ACS. The goals of decompressive laparotomy include decrease of increased IAP to stop organ dysfunction, allow for continued expansion of abdominal viscera during ongoing resuscitation, provide temporary abdominal coverage until the disease process resolves, prevent fascial retraction, and allow a means for continued evacuation of fluid. It is imperative that a complete fasciotomy of the abdominal wall is performed. The degree to which IAP decreases is a function of the degree to which the fascia is released. With decompression, there is an immediate decrease in IAP; however, the pressure may not decrease to normal levels. There should be an immediate recovery of some organ dysfunction (high respiratory pressures, hypotension) but the renal dysfunction may persist and require additional time to resolve.

Management of the resulting open abdomen is discussed later.

Summary

ACS is a life-threatening and treatable disease that requires a high index of suspicion to make the diagnosis before the onset of organ failure and prompt treatment once the diagnosis is made. The diagnosis of IAH is made using bladder pressure measurements in critically ill patients with known risk factors. Decompressive laparotomy is the treatment of choice in patients with intractable IAH or ACS.

Damage Control

Overall, about 10% to 15% of all laparotomies for trauma are managed with damage-control techniques.[1] In the past, damage control has been advocated in patients with exhaustion of physiologic reserves and imminent irreversible shock and death (patient in extremis), in cases with bleeding from difficult anatomic areas or complex injuries not amendable to easy surgical control, and for temporary stabilization and transfer to higher levels of care. Some investigators suggest that damage control should be considered in all patients in extremis, as defined by coagulopathy, hypothermia (<35°C), and severe acidosis with base deficit greater than 15 mmol/L. However, there is evidence that initiation of damage control before the patient becomes coagulopathic and in extremis improves survival.[2]

In summary, damage control should be considered early, before the patient reaches the extremis stage, taking into account the available resources, the nature of the injuries, the experience of the surgeon, the clinical condition of the patient, and any comorbid conditions. Major vascular injuries may be managed by temporary arterial shunting or venous ligation. Persistent bleeding from complex liver injuries, the retroperitoneum, or the pelvis may be managed by direct packing. Interventional angioembolization may be a useful adjunct to damage-control procedures, during surgery in hybrid operating rooms, or immediately after surgery in the angiography suite. Details of damage-control principles and techniques are outside the scope of this article. Following damage control, the fascia or the skin should never be closed, in order to increase the tamponade effect of packing, because most of these patients develop IAH. The abdomen should always be closed temporarily using one of the available materials and techniques.

Intra-abdominal Sepsis

The role of the open abdomen in the management of severe secondary peritonitis has been a controversial issue. In the 1980s and 1990s, from small retrospective studies, there was a significant interest and enthusiasm in the concept of treating severe peritonitis with the open-abdomen technique, using passive dressings for temporary abdominal closure.[3,4] However, subsequent studies failed to show any significant benefit. In a prospective, open, nonrandomized trial, sponsored by the Surgical Infection Society, 239 patients with surgical infection in the abdomen were treated with either the open-abdomen technique or laparotomy on demand. There was no significant difference in mortality between patients treated with a closed-abdomen technique (31% mortality) and those treated with variations of the open-abdomen technique (44% mortality).[5] In a 2007 study, Robledo and colleagues,[6] randomized 40 patients with severe secondary peritonitis into a open-abdomen group and a laparotomy-on-demand group. Although the difference in the mortalities between the open technique and laparotomy on demand (55% vs 30%) did not reach statistical significance, the relative risk and odds ratio for death were 1.83 and 2.85 times higher in the open-abdomen group. The study concluded that closed management of the abdomen may be a more rational approach in the management of severe peritonitis.

In summary, there is reasonable clinical evidence that temporary closure of the open abdomen using traditional abdominal packing is of no benefit and might be associated with increased mortality and a higher incidence of enteroatmospheric fistulas compared with the closed-abdomen and relaparotomy-on-demand technique.

However, recent experimental and clinical work has suggested that the open-abdomen technique with temporary abdominal wall closure using negative pressure therapy (NPT) methods is associated with superior outcomes. Amin and Shaikh,[7] in a prospective analysis of 20 patients requiring NPT following laparotomy for severe peritonitis, reported 100% survival. The study concluded that NPT is safe, but further studies are needed.

Horwood and colleagues,[8] in a study of 27 patients who were treated with an open abdomen and NPT, reported a significantly improved observed survival compared with P-POSSUM (physiological and operative severity score for the enumeration of mortality and morbidity) expected survival ($P = .004$). The study concluded that laparostomy with immediate NPT is a robust and effective system to manage patients with severe peritonitis.

Kubiak and colleagues,[9] in an experimental porcine model with intestinal ischemia/reperfusion and peritoneal fecal contamination, showed that the open abdomen combined with NPT (125 mm Hg) reduced mortality and organ dysfunction compared with animals treated with the traditional passive drainage. NPT removed significantly more peritoneal fluid, reduced systemic inflammation, and improved the histopathology in the intestine, lung, liver, and kidney.

In summary, the open abdomen has a major therapeutic role in damage-control procedures and in the management of IAH. There is some strong experimental and class III clinical evidence that the open abdomen with temporary closure using negative pressure techniques might be beneficial in the management of severe secondary peritonitis.

COMPLICATIONS OF THE OPEN ABDOMEN

Although the open abdomen has solved some serious and potentially lethal problems and has saved many lives, it is also associated with significant complications, such as major fluid and protein loss, nutritional problems, infections, loss of abdominal wall domain, large incisional hernias, and the development of enteroatmospheric fistulas.

The most effective way to prevent or reduce these complications is to close the abdominal wall as soon as possible, ideally within 5 to 7 days. Burlew and colleagues,[10] in a Western Trauma Association multiinstitutional study of 204 patients with enteric injuries managed with an open abdomen, found that fascia closure after day 5 had a 4 times higher likelihood of developing leak (3% vs 12%; $P = .02$). There is good evidence that, by using a strategy of avoiding excessive fluid resuscitation, application of effective temporary abdominal wall closure, and use of biological materials for fascia closure, definitive abdominal wall closure may be achieved earlier and at a higher rate.

TEMPORARY ABDOMINAL WALL CLOSURE

The technique used for temporary abdominal wall closure can influence outcomes, including survival, complications and success rate, and time to definitive fascia closure. The ideal method of temporary abdominal closure should prevent evisceration, actively remove any infected or toxic fluid from the peritoneal cavity, prevent the formation of enteroatmospheric fistulas, preserve the fascia and the abdominal wall domain, make reoperation easy and safe, and achieve early definitive closure.

Numerous materials and techniques have been used for temporary closure during the last decade, including skin approximation with towel clips or running suture, the Bogota bag, the Wittmann patch, absorbable synthetic meshes, and various NPT techniques (**Box 2**). Each technique has its own advantages and disadvantages:

- Skin approximation with towel clips or running suture has been suggested as a method for quick abdominal closure in damage-control procedures in patients in extremis. This type of closure is associated with an unacceptably high incidence of IAH and ACS and should not be used.[11,12]
- The Bogota bag or silo usually consists of a 3-L sterile irrigation bag or a sterile radiographic cassette cover, stapled or sutured to the fascia or the skin. It prevents evisceration of the abdominal contents while preventing or treating IAH or ACS. It is still used extensively in many countries because it is cheap, immediately available, and easy to apply. It might be valuable in cases with damage control for intra-abdominal bleeding in which definitive abdominal closure is anticipated within the next 2 or 3 days. However, it has now been abandoned by most modern trauma centers in the United States because of the development of new, more effective methods. Its major disadvantage is that it does not allow the effective removal of any infected or toxin-rich and cytokine-rich intraperitoneal fluid, and it does not prevent the loss of abdominal wall domain (**Fig. 1**).
- Absorbable or nonabsorbable meshes or sheets have been used for temporary abdominal wall closure. The material is sutured between the fascial edges and, as the bowel edema subsides, the mesh or sheet may be plicated and reduced in size, allowing gradual reapproximation of the fascia. Absorbable meshes may be left in place at the closure of the abdomen, whereas nonabsorbable materials usually need to be removed. If fascia or skin closure is not possible, usually

---

Box 2
Techniques for temporary abdominal wall closure

1. Skin approximation with towel clips or running suture

2. Bogota bag

3. Synthetic meshes

4. Velcro or zipper-type synthetic materials (Wittmann patch, Starsurgical)

5. Negative pressure dressing

    a. Vacuum pack (Barker technique)

    b. Vacuum-assisted closure (VAC Therapy, KCI)

    c. ABThera system (KCI)

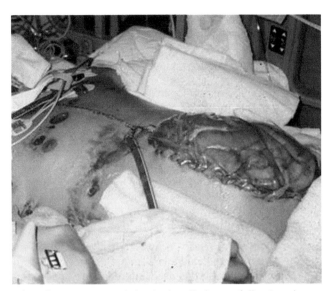

Fig. 1. Bogota bag for temporary abdominal wall closure following damage control for multiple gunshot wounds. It has limited or no role in the management of the open abdomen, especially in the presence of sepsis. It does not allow effective drainage of intra-abdominal toxin-rich fluid, does not reduce bowel edema, and does not preserve the wall domain.

because of persistent sepsis, the wound is allowed to granulate and is skin grafted at a later stage. This technique does not drain effectively any infected or toxic intra-abdominal fluid, it cannot be used in the presence of abdominal sepsis, it is associated with a high incidence of enteroatmospheric fistulas, parts of the mesh are often extruded, and there is a high incidence of incisional hernia (**Fig. 2**). The mesh traction technique, with gradual plication and approximation, might be combined with NPT and some studies have reported high primary fascia closure rates.[13–17]

- The Wittmann patch is another technique for temporary abdominal closure. The two opposite Velcro sheets are sutured to the fascial edges. The sheets overlap in the middle and allow gradual reapproximation of the fascia (**Fig. 3**). This technique preserves the abdominal wall domain but it does not allow effective drainage of any intra-abdominal infected fluid and is contraindicated in the presence of sepsis. In addition, there is concern that the sutures on the fascia might cause ischemic damage to the edges of the fascia, making the definitive closure operation more difficult. Some retrospective studies have shown a primary fascia closure rate of higher than 80%.[18] The Wittmann patch technique may be combined with NPT and there is some clinical evidence that, in the absence of sepsis, it increases the primary fascia rate.[19]
- NPT techniques have revolutionized the management of the open abdomen and improved survival, morbidity, and the success rate of primary fascia closure. This method prevents adhesions between the peritoneum and the bowel, preserves the abdominal wall domain, and actively drains toxin-rich or bacteria-rich intraperitoneal fluid. The 3 most commonly used NPT techniques are the Barker vacuum-pack technique, the vacuum-assisted closure (VAC; KCI, San Antonio, TX), and the ABThera (KCI, San Antonio, TX).

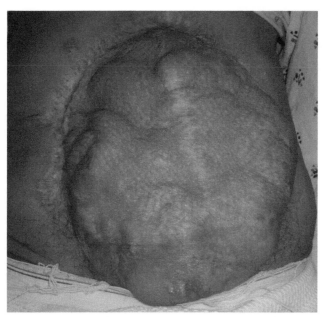

Fig. 2. Absorbable mesh for temporary abdominal wall closure: Subsequent skin grafting may be applied for wound cover but it results in incisional hernia.

○ The first negative pressure method for temporary abdominal wall closure was described in South Africa by Schein and colleagues[20] in 1986. The investigators described a sandwich technique composed of Marlex mesh and OpSite closure with suction catheters. This technique was modified by Barker and colleagues[21] in 1995 and was coined vacuum pack and later the Barker vacuum pack. The technique is simple and easily available. It consists of a fenestrated, nonadherent polyethylene sheet that is placed over the bowel and under the peritoneum, covered by moist surgical towels or gauze, 2 large silicone drains placed over the towels, and a transparent adhesive drape over the wound to maintain a closed seal. The drains are connected to continuous wall suction at 100 to

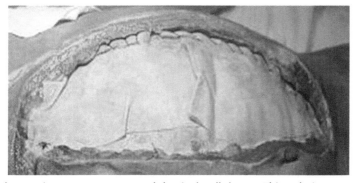

Fig. 3. Velcro or zipper-type temporary abdominal wall closure. This technique preserves the abdominal wall domain and facilitates fascia closure. It should not be used in the presence of sepsis. It may be combined with a negative pressure dressing.

150 mm Hg (**Fig. 4**). The dressing system is changed every 24 to 48 hours and every time the fascia at the top and bottom of the wound is approximated, if it can be done without tension. Some surgeons use this technique for the first 24 to 48 hours after surgery, switching to the VAC therapy afterward.

- The VAC Abdominal Dressing system (KCI) is a commercially available, sophisticated negative pressure dressing system that includes polyurethane foam covered with a protective, fenestrated, nonadherent layer, tubing, a canister, and a computerized pump (**Fig. 5**). The system pulls the fascia edges together and prevents adhesions between the bowel and anterior abdominal wall, making subsequent reexploration of the abdomen and fascia closure easier and safer. In addition, it actively removes any infected or inflammatory fluid from the peritoneal cavity.
- In 2009, a new generation of NPT, ABThera (KCI), received US Food and Drug Administration approval. This device consists of a visceral protective layer made of polyurethane foam with 6 radiating foam extensions enveloped in a polyethylene sheet with small fenestrations. This layer is placed directly over the bowel and tucked under the peritoneum, into the paracolic gutters and pelvis. The second layer consists of fenestrated foam cut into size and shape and placed over the protective foam, under the peritoneum. The third layer consists of a similar piece of foam placed over the previous layer, between the fascia edges. The dressing is then covered with a semiocclusive adhesive drape. A small piece of the adhesive drape and underlying sponge are excised and an interface pad with a tubing system is applied over this defect and connected to a NPT unit. The negative pressure collapses the foam, exerting

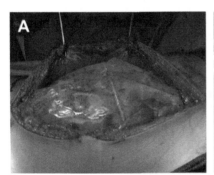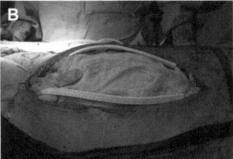

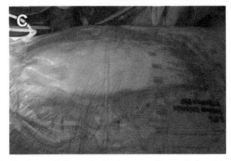

Fig. 4. Vacuum-pack technique. A fenestrated, nonadherent sheet is placed over the bowel and underneath the peritoneum (*A*), followed by moist surgical gauze and 2 drains (*B*), and then covered with a transparent adhesive dressing (*C*). The drains are connected to continuous wall suction (100–150 mm Hg).

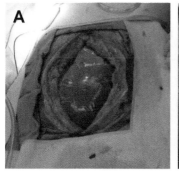
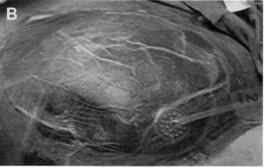

Fig. 5. (*A, B*) Abdominal VAC device.

medial traction and approximation of the fascia and abdominal wall. A pump canister collects and quantifies the fluid evacuated from the abdomen. Dressing changes are usually done every 2 to 3 days (**Fig. 6**).

The 3 main NPT modalities (Barker, VAC Abdominal Dressing system, ABThera) have different mechanical properties, which may affect outcomes. The most important difference is the distribution pattern of the preset negative pressure. In an experimental study, Sammons and colleagues[22] applied negative pressure of 125 mm Hg on a Barker system, VAC Abdominal Dressing system, and the ABThera system and measured the pressures at different areas of the dressing. In the Barker system the measured pressure at the center was reduced to 9 mm Hg and in the periphery it was only 2 mm Hg. In the VAC Abdominal Dressing, these numbers were 43 and 12 mm Hg, and in the ABThera system they were 88 and 71 mm Hg respectively (**Fig. 7A–C**). This distribution had a significant effect on the efficiency of the system in removing intraperitoneal fluid. In an animal model, Lindstedt and colleagues[23] found that the ABThera system was significantly more effective in removing peritoneal fluid and contracting the open abdomen than the VAC Abdominal Dressing.

The efficacy of the NPT system in removing infected or inflammatory peritoneal fluid may play a critical role in determining outcomes. Experimental work using a swine model of intestinal ischemia and peritoneal fecal contamination showed that early application of NPT with VAC Abdominal Dressing prevented the development of IAH and subsequent multi organ dysfunction syndrome (MODS) compared with treatment with passive drainage.[9] The suggested mechanism of protection was the effective removal of the peritoneal fluid containing inflammatory mediators, as shown by the reduction of the concentration of cytokines in the bloodstream.

The effect of NPT on the bowel is not known. There is concern that excessive negative pressure on the bowel surface may increase the risk of bowel fistula formation. There is experimental evidence that, with the ABThera system, there is little negative pressure transmitted directly to the bowel. In an animal model, Bjarnason and colleagues[17] studied the distribution of pressures after application of negative pressure settings of −50, −75, −100, −125, and −150 mm Hg with the ABThera system. The observed pressures within the 3 layers of foam correlated with the pressure settings. However, the median pressure at the bowel surface was between −2 and −10 mm Hg, regardless of pressure settings.

The optimal therapeutic negative pressure that stimulates cell reproduction and maximizes the tissue expansion effect is about 125 mm Hg. However, this pressure should be individualized. In cases with concerns about incomplete hemostasis, application of high negative pressures may aggravate the bleeding. In these cases, an initial

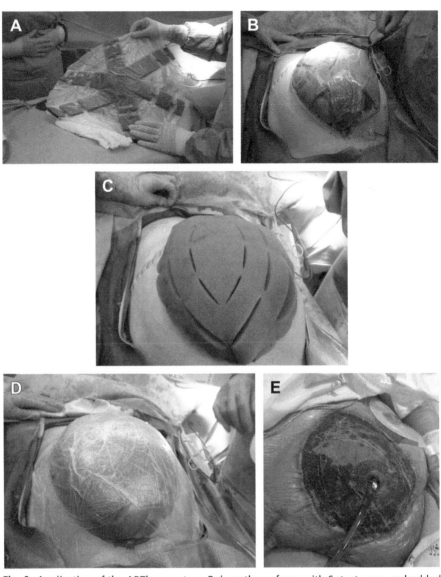

Fig. 6. Application of the ABThera system. Polyurethane foam with 6 strut arms, embedded between 2 fenestrated nonadherent sheets (*A*). It is placed directly over the bowel and tucked under the peritoneum (*B*). Perforated foam cut into size and shape is placed over the protective foam (*C*). The foam is covered by a semiocclusive adhesive drape (*D*). A small piece of the adhesive drape and underlying sponge is excised and an interface pad with a tubing system is applied over this opening and connected to a NPT unit (*E*).

low negative pressure is advisable. If large amounts of frank blood are seen in the canister of the vacuum pump, the negative pressure should immediately be discontinued and the patient returned to the operating room for reexploration and bleeding control. In addition, although rare, IAH may occur in some cases with temporary abdominal wall closure. It is important that, after surgery, the amount of bleeding in the NPT canister is measured continuously. Also, the bladder pressure should

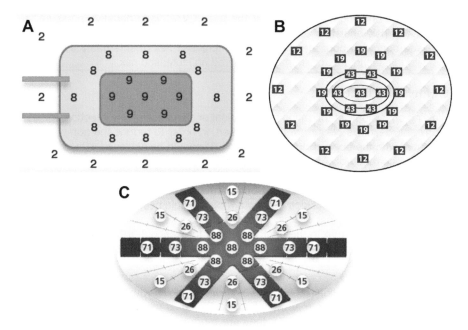

Fig. 7. Application of -125 mm Hg. Distribution of negative pressures in vacuum pack, VAC Abdominal Dressing and ABThera techniques. Note the even distribution of pressures in AB-Thera (*C*) and the uneven distribution in the vacuum pack (*A*) and VAC (*B*). (*Data from* Sammons A, Delgado A, Cheatham M. Clinical symposium on advances in skin and wound care. San Antonio (TX): 2009.)

be monitored routinely during the first few hours of negative pressure dressing application.

Comparison of Techniques for Temporary Abdominal Closure

In a systematic review of the literature, Quyn and colleagues[19] compared different methods of temporary abdominal closure, including Bogota bag, dynamic retention sutures, zipper, Wittmann patch, and VAC. The new generation of NPT device, ABThera, was not included. The investigators concluded that, in the absence of sepsis, Wittmann patch and VAC Abdominal Dressing offered the best outcome. In the presence of sepsis, VAC had the highest delayed primary closure and the lowest mortality. However, the investigators stressed that, because of data heterogeneity, only limited conclusions could be drawn from the analysis.

Some investigators combined VAC with the Bogota bag[24] and others the VAC with mesh[15] with good results.

In a recent prospective, observational, open-label parallel study, Cheatham and colleagues[25] compared the Barker vacuum-pack technique with the ABThera NPT system (KCI USA, Inc, San Antonio, TX) in 280 patients requiring open-abdomen management. The 2 study groups were well matched demographically. Thirty-day primary fascia closure rate was 69% for ABThera and 51% for Barker ($P = .03$). The all-cause mortality was 14% and 30% respectively ($P = .01$). Multivariate regression analysis showed that patients treated with ABThera were significantly more likely to survive compared with patients treated with Barker (odds ratio, 3.17; 95% confidence interval, 1.22–8.26; $P = .02$) after controlling for age and severity of illness.

There is an ongoing debate whether the use of VAC, with negative pressure, increases the risk of fistula formation. Although some small retrospective studies expressed concern about the possibility of increased risk of enteroatmospheric fistulas with this technique, other studies showed no increased risk.[26,27]

DEFINITIVE FASCIA CLOSURE

Following physiologic stabilization of the patient or clearance of any infection, the goal is early and definitive closure of the abdomen, in order to reduce the complications associated with the open abdomen. The closure should be achieved without tension or risk of recurrence of IAH. Primary fascia closure may be possible in many cases within a few days of the initial operation, when any intra-abdominal packing is removed, the infection clears, and the bowel edema subsides. However, in many patients, early definitive fascial closure may not be possible because of persistent bowel edema or intra-abdominal sepsis. In these cases, progressive closure should be attempted at every return to the operating room for washout or dressing change, by placing a few interrupted sutures at the top and bottom of the fascia defect (**Fig. 8**).

In patients with persistent large fascial defects, definitive reconstruction has been described using synthetic or biologic meshes or sheets, or autologous tissue transfer with component separation. In choosing materials, bridging with biologics is preferred, especially if there is concern about infection. Biologics have numerous advantages compared with synthetic materials: they are more resistant to infection, if they get infected there is no need to be removed, and in the long term they maintain a satisfactory tensile strength. However, long-term studies are still lacking and the durability of the different biologic meshes has not been clinically proved. Early biologic materials (Alloderm, Lifecell) resulted in herniation or mesh laxity in up to 100% of cases.[28] Advances in biologics have improved the quality and durability of the new meshes, and more recent studies describe much lower rates. However, the long-term durability of the different biologic meshes used to close the open abdomen is still unknown.[29–31] Acellular matrix materials, prepared from cadaver or animal skin or animal intestine, are commercially available. Every attempt should be made to cover the prosthetic material with skin, in order to decrease the risk of infection and fistula formation. This coverage can almost always be achieved by undermining skin flaps, up to the anterior axillary lines bilaterally. If skin coverage is not possible, application of negative pressure therapy over the prosthetic material and subsequent skin grafting of the granulation tissue may be considered, although the effect of NPT on the integrity of the exposed biologic mesh has not been adequately explored.

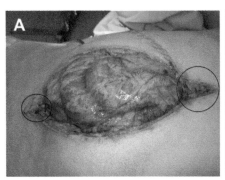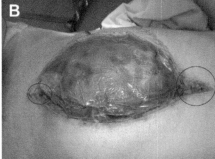

Fig. 8. (*A, B*) Progressive closure of the upper and lower parts of the incision 24 hours after the initial application of ABThera (*circles*).

Enteroatmospheric Fistulas

The development of enteroatmospheric fistulas is the most serious and challenging local complication in an open abdomen. The overall incidence of this complication is about 5%.[32,33] However, in the chronically open abdomen, the incidence increases to about 15%.[34] The exposed bowel is at risk of fistulization if the abdomen remains open for longer than 5 to 7 days, especially in the presence of synthetic meshes or infection. There is an ongoing debate whether the use of NPT increases the risk of fistulization. Although some small retrospective studies expressed concern about the possibility of increased risk of enteroatmospheric fistulas with NPT, other studies showed no increased risk.[26,30,35] The issue is still unresolved and better studies are needed to address this concern.

The development of an enteroatmospheric fistula increases the ICU stay by 3-fold, the hospital stay by 4-fold, and the hospital charges by 4.5-fold (**Table 1**).[34] In some cases, numerous enteroatmospheric fistulas may develop, and the constant leak of enteric contents on the open abdomen aggravates the inflammation and encourages the formation of new fistulas (**Fig. 9**). The most effective way of preventing this catastrophic complication is early closure of the abdominal wall. The management strategy should include temporary local control to prevent spillage of enteric contents on the surrounding tissues, while planning the definitive closure of the fistula.

Local control of the enteroatmospheric fistula

Local control of the enteroatmospheric fistula is difficult because it is not possible to apply an ostomy bag. The leak of intestinal contents on the surrounding exposed bowel or granulation tissue, the chemical irritation of the skin, and the soiling and malodor create a challenging task for the physicians and nurses and a distressing situation for the patient.

Efforts to create a controlled fistula by inserting a Foley catheter never succeed and they usually make the fistula larger (**Fig. 10**). Attempts to suture the fistula rarely succeed, unless the repair is immediately covered by normal skin or skin graft.

Appropriate use of the VAC system may be helpful in many cases. Sometimes, especially in small fistulas, the negative pressure approximates the edges of the fistula and spontaneous closure may occur, The VAC system may allow a controlled diversion of the fistula contents, protect the surrounding open abdomen and normal skin, and provide comfort to the patient from the chemical dermatitis pain, odor, and soilage.

Different VAC techniques may be used to achieve controlled diversion of the effluent, depending on the nature of enteric contents. In thin, liquid contents, the VAC technique includes (1) a single layer of petroleum-based fine mesh gauze placed over the wound bed, leaving the fistula uncovered. (2) The VAC WhiteFoam is cut to

Table 1			
Effect of fistula formation on hospital resources			
	Fistula	**No Fistula**	**P Value**
ICU days	25.7	8.8	.02
Hospital days	82.5	20.0	<.01
Hospital charges ($)	514,758	112,508	<.001

Thirty-six patients with fistulas matched to 36 controls (matched for age, gender, mechanism, injury severity score (ISS), Glasgow coma score (GCS), damage-control laparotomy).

Data from Teixeira PG, Inaba K, Dubose J, et al. Enterocutaneous fistula complicating trauma laparotomy: a major resource burden. Am Surg 2009;75(1):30–2.

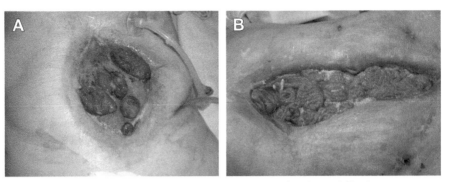

Fig. 9. (*A, B*) Local control of multiple enteroatmospheric fistulae is difficult.

size 1 to 2 cm larger than the mouth of the fistula and placed directly over the fistula. (3) The VAC GranuFoam is cut to size to cover the remaining wound, leaving an opening around the WhiteFoam. (4) An adhesive transparent drape is applied over the sponge. (5) A 2-cm to 2.5-cm opening is made on the transparent drape and the superficial part of the WhiteFoam is excised, directly over the fistula. A thin layer of the foam still covers the fistula. (6) An interface pad with a tubing system is applied over the opening and connected to a NPT unit (**Fig. 11**). The level of negative pressure should be individualized and adjusted over the next few days, aiming for the lowest output without effluent leak around the stoma. In some patients, high negative pressures increase the fistula output, whereas in others it reduces the output by approximating the edges of the fistula.

Another method described to control fistulas with watery output is the nipple technique.[36] This technique uses a standard baby bottle nipple of latex or silicone over the fistula. A hole of approximately 3 to 4 mm is cut in the tip of the nipple, through which a Malecot or Foley catheter with a slightly inflated balloon is inserted and positioned in the apex of the nipple so as to prevent direct contact with the bowel (**Fig. 12**). A nonadherent, petroleum jelly–impregnated gauze is then placed over the rest of the bowel.

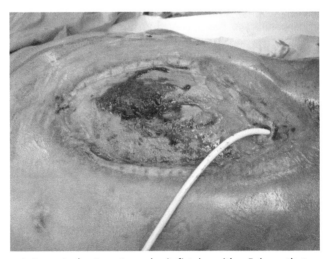

Fig. 10. Attempts to control enteroatmospheric fistulas with a Foley catheter are futile and make the fistula bigger.

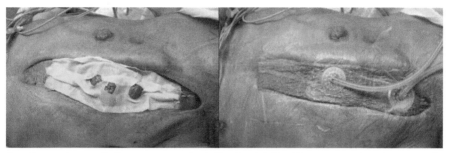

Fig. 11. Local control of enteroatmospheric fistula with liquid contents, using the VAC technique (described in the text).

In addition, an abdominal wound VAC sponge is cut to size and shape to fit the open abdomen, adhesive drape is applied, and a small hole is cut in it to accommodate the nipple with the catheter. VAC suction is then applied at 125 mm Hg and the fistula catheter is placed to gravity drainage.

The systems described earlier work well with proximal intestinal fistulas with watery effluent. In more solid intestinal contents, the system clogs and does not drain effectively. In these cases, different techniques, such as the fistula ring,[37] may be useful for temporary control of the enteric contents.

The fistula ring technique involves the following steps: (1) a round piece of foam, about 3 to 4 cm larger than the fistula, is cut into a ring with a diameter about 2 cm bigger than the fistula. (2) The ring is sandwiched with adhesive drape. An Eakin ring is applied at the base of the ring. If needed, 1 or 2 small holes are made on the lateral surface of the ring to allow negative pressure to reduce the overall height of the ring. (3) A small hole is created in the drape, the size of the fistula, in the middle of the ring. (4) A single layer of petroleum-based fine mesh gauze is placed over the

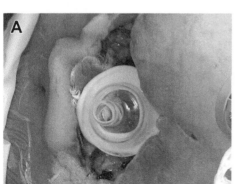
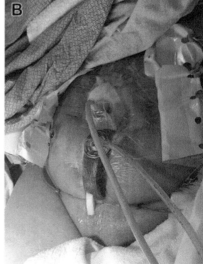

Fig. 12. (*A, B*) The nipple technique may be useful in selected enteroatmospheric fistulae with liquid contents.

open abdomen, leaving the fistula uncovered. (5) The ring is applied over the fistula. (6) The GranuFoam is cut to a size and shape to fit the abdominal wound, placed on the wound bed around the ring, and covered with an adhesive drape. (7) An interface pad with a tubing system is applied, not close to the fistula, and NPT of 100 to 125 mm Hg is initiated. (8) An ostomy bag is then applied over the ring to collect the effluent (**Fig. 13**).

The role of somatostatin administration is not clear. In a meta-analysis of 9 randomized controlled trials, Rahbour and colleagues[38] concluded that somatostatin analogues seem to decrease the duration of enterocutaneous fistulas and duration of hospital stay, but no mortality benefit was identified. There are no studies on the role of somatostatin in the management of enteroatmospheric fistulas, and it is not known whether the results with enterocutaneous fistulas can be extrapolated to enteroatmospheric fistulas. It might be useful to administer somatostatin in high-output fistulas and continue treatment only if there is a significant reduction of the effluent.

Surgical Management of Enteroatmospheric Fistulas

Although some small, low-output fistulas may close spontaneously with the help with NPT, most need surgical repair. The nutritional status of the patient is a critical factor in determining the outcome of the surgical repair of the fistula. Total parenteral nutrition is the basis of the nutritional support of the patient, although for distal, low-output fistulas, some enteral nutrition may be possible. No major operation should be undertaken if the nutritional status of the patient is poor, as reflected by low prealbumin levels.

The operative management of the enteroatmospheric fistulas is a major technical challenge and ideally these cases should be referred to centers with significant experience in the management of this problem. There are different surgical options, depending on the site, size, and shape of the fistula and the experience of the surgeon.

A

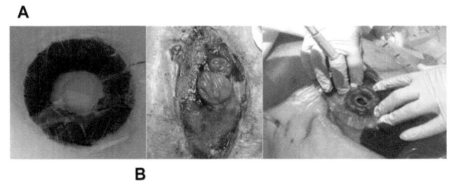

B

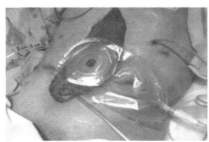

Fig. 13. (*A, B*) The fistula ring technique may be useful in difficult enteroatmospheric fistulae, including those with thick contents.

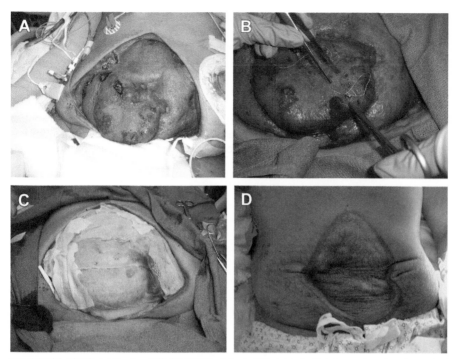

Fig. 14. (*A–D*) Closure of multiple, small enteroatmospheric fistulae using local surgical repair. (*B*) Local debridement and closure with absorbable suture. (*C*) The open abdomen is covered with thin skin graft. (*D*) The result many weeks later.

The options may range from local closure of the fistula to highly complex and risky abdominal exploration and bowel excision.

In some cases with small fistulas, local debridement, repair with fine absorbable sutures, and immediate coverage with mobilized skin flaps or coverage with skin graft is

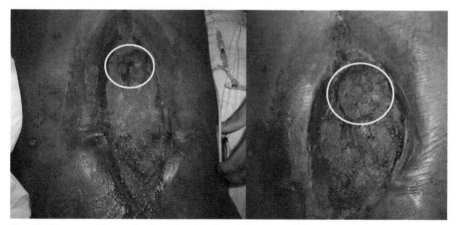

Fig. 15. Closure of large fistula, using local mobilization of the involved small bowel loop, debridement, and repair of the fistula. The repair should always be covered with mobilized skin flaps or skin graft. Circle on left side shows the fistula and on the right side it shows the closed and grafted fistula.

usually successful (**Fig. 14**A–D). Failure to cover the repair with the patient's own tissues will almost certainly result in breakdown of the repair. Use of biologic dressings to cover the wound is not as effective and should not be considered.

In patients with large and retracted fistula openings, local mobilization of the involved small bowel loop, debridement, and repair of the fistula may be possible (**Fig. 15**). This procedure should be done with the help of magnifying loupes. The wound is then covered with mobilized skin flaps or skin graft, as described earlier. Even if the repair breaks down, the grafted tissues around the fistula make the control of the effluent easier with an easy application of an ostomy bag. In addition, it stops the fluid and protein losses from the open wound and reduces the risk of more fistula formation.

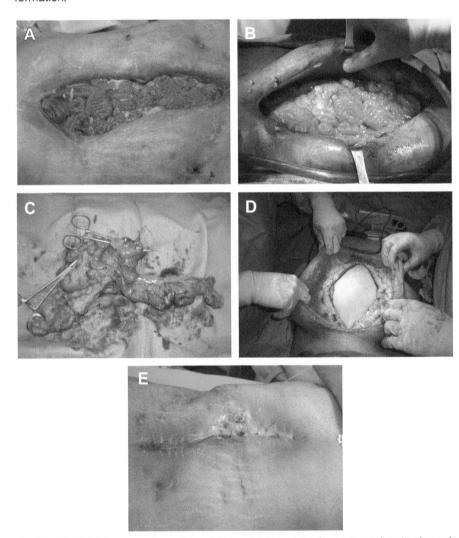

Fig. 16. (A) Multiple enteroatmospheric fistulae. (B) Entry into the peritoneal cavity through the lateral edge of the wound. (C) Resection of the segment of bowel containing the fistulae. (D) Closure of the fascia with biologic material and mobilization of the skin flaps bilaterally. (E) Postoperative results.

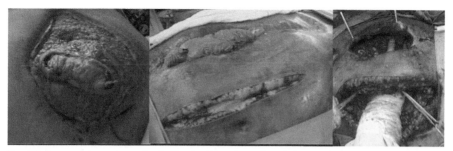

Fig. 17. Large enteroatmospheric fistula. Entry into the abdomen through the edge of the wound was not possible. Entry into the peritoneal cavity through a lateral incision was successful.

In patients with large fistulas and retracted stomas, or in the presence of distal obstruction, local repair of the fistula is not possible. In these cases, exploratory laparotomy with resection of the involved bowel loop and anastomosis remain the only option. Any major operation should be delayed for 4 to 6 months, if possible, to allow inflammation and edema to subside, and to improve the patient's nutritional status. Use of a headlight and magnifying loupes make the dissection of the tissues easier and safer. Entry into the peritoneal cavity should first be attempted through the lateral edge of the wound (**Fig. 16**). If this is not possible because of the often frozen and hostile anterior abdomen, entry may be attempted through a lateral incision, away from the open wound.[39] A long vertical incision is performed approximately 8 to 10 cm lateral to the open abdominal wound. The peritoneum in that area is usually free of difficult adhesions and entry into the peritoneal cavity is easy (**Fig. 17**). Mobilization of the bowel is achieved under direct vision, posterolaterally, and the matted mass of bowel loops lying under the granulation tissue of the abdominal wound is then resected en masse and the continuity of the small bowel is reestablished. The fascia defect is closed with a biologic material. The skin and subcutaneous tissue are then mobilized at the fascia level, up to the anterior axillary lines, and the skin is closed over 2 drains. The drains should be kept for several days until they are almost completely dry. Use of tissue expanders or complex abdominal flaps is not necessary and they are often associated with serious complications and failure.

SUMMARY

The open abdomen has become the standard of care in damage-control procedures, the management of IAH, and in severe intra-abdominal sepsis. This approach has saved many lives but has also created new problems, such as severe fluid and protein loss, nutritional problems, enteroatmospheric fistulas, fascial retraction with loss of abdominal domain, and development of massive incisional hernias. Early definitive closure is the basis of preventing or reducing the risk of these complications. The introduction of new techniques and materials for temporary and subsequent definitive abdominal closure has improved outcomes in this group of patients.

REFERENCES

1. Teixeira PG, Salim A, Inaba K, et al. A prospective look at the current state of open abdomens. Am Surg 2008;74(10):891–7.

2. Hirshberg A, Wall MJ Jr, Mattox KL. Planned reoperation for trauma: a two year experience with 124 consecutive patients. J Trauma 1994;37(3):365–9.

3. Guthy E. Surgical aspects in the management of peritonitis. Scand J Gastroenterol Suppl 1984;100:49–52.

4. Hedderich GS, Wexler MJ, McLean AP, et al. The septic abdomen: open management with Marlex mesh with a zipper. Surgery 1986;99(4):399–408.

5. Christou NV, Barie PS, Dellinger EP, et al. Surgical infection society intra-abdominal infection study. Prospective evaluation of management techniques and outcome. Arch Surg 1993;128(2):193–8 [discussion: 198–9].

6. Robledo FA, Luque-de-Leon E, Suarez R, et al. Open versus closed management of the abdomen in the surgical treatment of severe secondary peritonitis: a randomized clinical trial. Surg Infect (Larchmt) 2007;8(1):63–72.

7. Amin AI, Shaikh IA. Topical negative pressure in managing severe peritonitis: a positive contribution? World J Gastroenterol 2009;15(27):3394–7.

8. Horwood J, Akbar F, Maw A. Initial experience of laparostomy with immediate vacuum therapy in patients with severe peritonitis. Ann R Coll Surg Engl 2009; 91(8):681–7.

9. Kubiak BD, Albert SP, Gatto LA, et al. Peritoneal negative pressure therapy prevents multiple organ injury in a chronic porcine sepsis and ischemia/reperfusion model. Shock 2010;34(5):525–34.

10. Burlew CC, Moore EE, Cuschieri J, et al. Sew it up! A Western Trauma Association multi-institutional study of enteric injury management in the postinjury open abdomen. J Trauma 2011;70(2):273–7.

11. Offner PJ, de Souza AL, Moore EE, et al. Avoidance of abdominal compartment syndrome in damage-control laparotomy after trauma. Arch Surg 2001;136(6):676–81.

12. Raeburn CD, Moore EE, Biffl WL, et al. The abdominal compartment syndrome is a morbid complication of postinjury damage control surgery. Am J Surg 2001; 182(6):542–6.

13. Dietz UA, Wichelmann C, Wunder C, et al. Early repair of open abdomen with a tailored two-component mesh and conditioning vacuum packing: a safe alternative to the planned giant ventral hernia. Hernia 2012;16(4):451–60.

14. Rasilainen SK, Mentula PJ, Leppaniemi AK. Vacuum and mesh-mediated fascial traction for primary closure of the open abdomen in critically ill surgical patients. Br J Surg 2012;99(12):1725–32.

15. Petersson U, Acosta S, Bjorck M. Vacuum-assisted wound closure and mesh-mediated fascial traction–a novel technique for late closure of the open abdomen. World J Surg 2007;31(11):2133–7.

16. Seternes A, Myhre HO, Dahl T. Early results after treatment of open abdomen after aortic surgery with mesh traction and vacuum-assisted wound closure. Eur J Vasc Endovasc Surg 2010;40(1):60–4.

17. Bjarnason T, Montgomery A, Hlebowicz J, et al. Pressure at the bowel surface during topical negative pressure therapy of the open abdomen: an experimental study in a porcine model. World J Surg 2011;35(4):917–23.

18. Tieu BH, Cho SD, Luem N, et al. The use of the Wittmann patch facilitates a high rate of fascial closure in severely injured trauma patients and critically ill emergency surgery patients. J Trauma 2008;65(4):865–70.

19. Quyn AJ, Johnston C, Hall D, et al. The open abdomen and temporary abdominal closure systems–historical evolution and systematic review. Colorectal Dis 2012; 14(8):e429–38.

20. Schein M, Saadia R, Jamieson JR, et al. The 'sandwich technique' in the management of the open abdomen. Br J Surg 1986;73(5):369–70.

21. Brock WB, Barker DE, Burns RP. Temporary closure of open abdominal wounds: the vacuum pack. Am Surg 1995;61(1):30–5.
22. Sammons A, Delgado A, Cheatham M. Clinical symposium on advances in skin and wound care. San Antonio (TX): 2009.
23. Lindstedt S, Malmsjo M, Hlebowicz J, et al. Comparative study of the microvascular blood flow in the intestinal wall, wound contraction and fluid evacuation during negative pressure wound therapy in laparostomy using the V.A.C. abdominal dressing and the ABThera open abdomen negative pressure therapy system. Int Wound J 2013. [Epub ahead of print].
24. Von Ruden C, Benninger E, Mayer D, et al. Bogota-VAC – a newly modified temporary abdominal closure technique. Eur J Trauma Emerg Surg 2008;34:582–6.
25. Cheatham ML, Demetriades D, Fabian TC, et al. A prospective study examining clinical outcomes associated with a negative pressure wound therapy system and Barker's vacuum packing technique. World J Surg 2013;37:2018–30.
26. Rao M, Burke D, Finan PJ, et al. The use of vacuum-assisted closure of abdominal wounds: a word of caution. Colorectal Dis 2007;9(3):266–8.
27. Shaikh IA, Ballard-Wilson A, Yalamarthi S, et al. Use of topical negative pressure in assisted abdominal closure does not lead to high incidence of enteric fistulae. Colorectal Dis 2010;12(9):931–4.
28. de Moya MA, Dunham M, Inaba K, et al. Long-term outcome of acellular dermal matrix when used for large traumatic open abdomen. J Trauma 2008;65(2): 349–53.
29. Shah BC, Tiwari MM, Goede MR, et al. Not all biologics are equal! Hernia 2011; 15(2):165–71.
30. Shaikh FM, Giri SK, Durrani S, et al. Experience with porcine acellular dermal collagen implant in one-stage tension-free reconstruction of acute and chronic abdominal wall defects. World J Surg 2007;31(10):1966–72 [discussion: 1973–4, 1975].
31. Janfaza M, Martin M, Skinner R. A preliminary comparison study of two noncrosslinked biologic meshes used in complex ventral hernia repairs. World J Surg 2012;36(8):1760–4.
32. Barker DE, Kaufman HJ, Smith LA, et al. Vacuum pack technique of temporary abdominal closure: a 7-year experience with 112 patients. J Trauma 2000; 48(2):201–6 [discussion: 206–7].
33. Smith LA, Barker DE, Chase CW, et al. Vacuum pack technique of temporary abdominal closure: a four-year experience. Am Surg 1997;63(12):1102–7 [discussion: 1107–8].
34. Teixeira PG, Inaba K, Dubose J, et al. Enterocutaneous fistula complicating trauma laparotomy: a major resource burden. Am Surg 2009;75(1):30–2.
35. Starr-Marshall K. Vacuum-assisted closure of abdominal wounds and enterocutaneous fistulae; the St Marks experience. Colorectal Dis 2007;9(6):573.
36. Layton B, Dubose J, Nichols S, et al. Pacifying the open abdomen with concomitant intestinal fistula: a novel approach. Am J Surg 2010;199(4):e48–50.
37. Goverman J, Yelon JA, Platz JJ, et al. The "fistula VAC," a technique for management of enterocutaneous fistulae arising within the open abdomen: report of 5 cases. J Trauma 2006;60(2):428–31 [discussion: 431].
38. Rahbour G, Siddiqui MR, Ullah MR, et al. A meta-analysis of outcomes following use of somatostatin and its analogues for the management of enterocutaneous fistulas. Ann Surg 2012;256(6):946–54.
39. Demetriades D. A technique of surgical closure of complex intestinal fistulae in the open abdomen. J Trauma 2003;55(5):999–1001.

Necrotizing Skin and Soft Tissue Infections

Haytham M.A. Kaafarani, MD, MPH*, David R. King, MD

KEYWORDS

- Necrotizing skin and soft tissue infection (NSSTI) • Necrotizing fasciitis
- Gas gangrene • Fournier's gangrene • Wide local debridement

KEY POINTS

- Necrotizing skin and soft tissue infections (NSSTIs) are caused by aggressive and often toxin-secreting bacteria.
- NSSTIs may be caused by single agents such as clostridia or streptococci (type I), but are often polymicrobial (type II).
- Immunosuppressed individuals are especially susceptible to NSSTIs.
- Systemic signs of infection are ubiquitous, with patients often becoming septic and showing signs of multiorgan dysfunction syndrome.
- The Laboratory Risk Indicator for Necrotizing Fasciitis has a high positive and negative predictive value for NSSTIs.
- Computed tomography might be helpful in diagnosing NSSTIs, but is often not sufficient to rule it out.
- Prompt wide surgical debridement and broad spectrum antibiotics are the key elements needed for successful management and prevention of the high morbidity and mortality associated with NSSTIs.

INTRODUCTION

Necrotizing skin and soft tissue infections (NSSTIs) are severe infections resulting in life-threatening soft tissue destruction and necrosis and resulting from toxin-secreting bacteria. Extensive, rapid, and widespread progression of the infection and necrosis along soft tissue planes is the essential characteristics of the disease.

Epidemiology

The epidemiology of NSSTIs is not very well established; reliable data on its incidence are largely absent from medical literature, and most published studies reflect

Division of Trauma, Emergency Surgery and Surgical Critical Care, Massachusetts General Hospital, Harvard Medical School, 165 Cambridge Street, Suite 810, Boston, MA 02114, USA
* Corresponding author.
E-mail address: hkaafarani@partners.org

Surg Clin N Am 94 (2014) 155–163
http://dx.doi.org/10.1016/j.suc.2013.10.011
0039-6109/14/$ – see front matter © 2014 Elsevier Inc. All rights reserved.

surgical.theclinics.com

individual institutional experiences. Using the Centers for Disease Control and Prevention data, O'Loughlin and colleagues[1] report an incidence of 3.5 cases in 100,000 persons of NSSTIs specifically caused by group A streptococcus in the United States and a case-fatality rate of 13.7%. Viewing the wide variation in reporting the clinical specifics, the treatment modalities, the outcome, and eventual prognosis of NSSTI patients, there is a definite need for large national multi-institutional registries for NSSTIs, similar to those existing for trauma or oncology patients.

History

One of the earlier medical references to NSSTIs was in 1871, whereby more than 2600 cases were reported during the American Civil War by a Confederate Army surgeon, Joseph Jones.[2] At that time and continuing until the early to mid 20th century, the disease entity was popularized in media as being caused by "flesh-eating bacteria," obviously a misnomer. NSSTI is also referred to in medical literature as gas gangrene, necrotizing skin and skin structure infections, necrotizing fasciitis, Fournier gangrene (when affecting the groin, genital organs, and perineum), and Ludwig angina (when affecting the submandibular floor of the mouth, usually in relationship with serious dental infections).

PATHOPHYSIOLOGY

Occasionally, an infection entry point such as a subtle wound is present on physical examination. The history of an insect bite or minor laceration can also be occasionally elicited. Many other times, such history or evidence of a wound break is not present.

Microbiology

There are 2 types of NSSTIs. Type I infections are monomicrobial and are most commonly caused by anaerobic bacteria such as clostridia, streptococci, or bacteroides species. Type II infections are polymicrobial in cause. Most causative pathogens, especially *Clostridium perfringens*, secrete exotoxins (eg, hemolysins, collagenases, lecithinases, proteases) that lead to fast evolution of deep tissue necrosis along fascial and muscle layers. Concomitant small-vessel thrombosis results in the grayish skin hue that is often noted on careful examination of these patients. Due to both the small vessel thrombosis and the progression of infection along deeper soft tissue layers, the infection is often more widespread than apparent on physical examination of the underlying skin. Systemically, the secreted exotoxins lead to increased cytokine production, T-cell proliferation, as well as interleukin (IL) and lymphokine secretion (IL-1, IL-2 IL-6, tumor necrosis factor-α and -β), clinically leading to severe sepsis/septic shock, pronounced systemic inflammatory response syndrome, and not uncommonly, multi-organ dysfunction syndrome.

Risk factors

Immunocompromised patients, including patients with diabetes mellitus, human immunodeficiency virus, malnutrition, peripheral vascular disease or malignancy, and intravenous drug abuse patients, are at an especially increased risk of developing NSSTIs.

CLINICAL MANIFESTATION

Early suspicion and prompt diagnosis of NSSTIs are critical, as fast progression to systemic shock and lethal septic shock are definite if aggressive control of the infection is not obtained.

Signs and Symptoms

Patients often complain of pain out of proportion to physical examination findings and report tenderness beyond the area of concern. Hemorrhagic skin bullae, grayish skin discoloration, and multiple blisters of different sizes are often present but are not specific findings to NSSTIs (**Fig. 1**). "Dishwasher-like" discharge from the area of concern is almost pathognomonic. Crepitus has been classically described, but is rarely present on examination nowadays. Patients often show signs of systemic toxicity with altered mental status, hypotension, and tachycardia.

Laboratory Workup

Laboratory workup typically reveals significant leukocytosis with marked left shift or even bandemia, serious metabolic disturbances, and multiple electrolyte imbalances, most commonly hyponatremia and acidosis. Creatine kinase levels are also often elevated. In cases of septic shock, creatinine clearance is compromised with early signs of acute renal failure. The Laboratory Risk Indicator for Necrotizing Fasciitis (LRI-NEC), a purely laboratory-based score, is one of several clinical tools available to help physicians and surgeons recognizing early-stage NSSTIs. Differentiating an early NSSTI from a more "benign" skin and soft tissue infection can be very challenging, but is crucial especially when considering the completely different treatment management strategies needed and the drastically different prognosis of each. LRINEC is an objective score based on 6 laboratory values (white blood cell count, hemoglobin, C-reactive protein, sodium, glucose, and creatinine levels) (**Table 1**). In the original validation study, an LRINEC score ≥6 had a positive predictive value of 92% and a negative predictive of 96% for NSSTI.[3] Subsequent attempts at validating LRINEC have failed to show reliable sensitivity.[4,5]

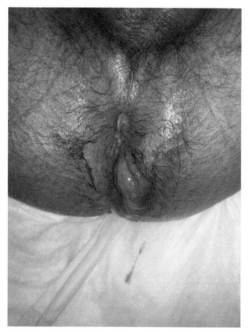

Fig. 1. Clinical presentation of necrotizing skin and soft tissue infection.

Table 1 The LRINEC	
Variable	Points
WBC count ($\times 10^6/mm^3$)	
<15	0
15–25	1
>25	2
Hemoglobin (g/dL)	
>13.5	0
11–13.5	1
<11	2
C-reactive protein >150 mg/L	4
Sodium (mmol/L) <135	2
Creatinine >141 umol/L	2
Glucose >10 mmol/L	1

Radiography

Plain films are rarely helpful because the presence of soft tissue air on radiograph has an extremely low sensitivity for NSSTIs. Computed tomography scan reveals soft tissue stranding and edema at the deeper fascial or muscular layers and occasionally will show gas between these tissue layers, even when the causative agent is not anaerobic or clostridial. The presence of gas on computed tomography scan is highly specific but, unfortunately, has a low sensitivity. Other radiologic signs suggesting NSSTI include nonhomogenous enhancement of muscle tissue by intravenous contrast and multiple noncontiguous fluid collections. Magnetic resonance imaging can be oversensitive, and the authors do not encourage its use to diagnose NSSTIs.

Surgical Exploration

Surgical exploration is the only reliable method to differentiate between benign soft tissue infection and NSSTIs. Intraoperatively, NSSTIs are characterized by pale or necrotic soft tissue/muscle/fascia, absence of abrupt bleeding on sharp tissue surgical dissection, "dishwasher-like" gray discharge, and effortless separation and elevation of tissue planes with easy finger "sliding" between the muscle and fascia layers, as well as between subcutaneous tissue and fascia layers (the "finger test").

TREATMENT

NSSTI is a surgical emergency and warrants immediate and aggressive treatment with simultaneous (1) hemodynamic support and fluid resuscitation, (2) wide surgical debridement, and (3) broad-spectrum antibiotics. Adjunctive treatment modalities include hyperbaric oxygen and intravenous immunoglobulins. Attempts at radiographic confirmation of the diagnosis should be deferred if they will delay the operative intervention.

Hemodynamic Support and Fluid Resuscitation

Many patients with NSSTIs are septic and show early signs of shock. It is recommended to treat them using the surviving sepsis guidelines[6] with early institution of intravenous antibiotics, fluid resuscitation to a central venous pressure of 8 to 12, a mean arterial pressure greater than 65 mm Hg, urine output greater than 0.5 mL/kg/h, and

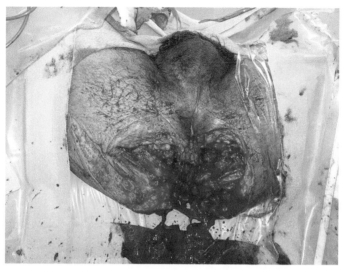

Fig. 2. Wide surgical debridement of necrotizing skin and soft tissue infection.

central or mixed venous oxygen saturation greater than 65% to 70%. If lactate levels were elevated, normalization of lactate levels with resuscitation should be sought. Vasopressors should be used early, as needed.

Wide Surgical Debridement

All necrotic tissue needs to be aggressively debrided until all remaining tissue is healthy, clearly viable, and bleeds briskly (**Figs. 2** and **3**). The overlying skin should always be resected irrespective of its appearance because of microscopic vessel thrombosis that will eventually lead to its necrosis, if not resected. Temporary dressing

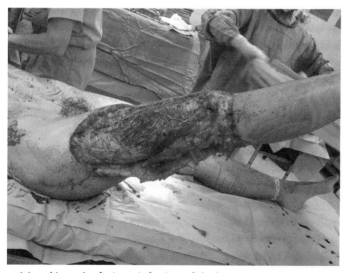

Fig. 3. Necrotizing skin and soft tissue infection of the lower extremity requiring serial wide debridement.

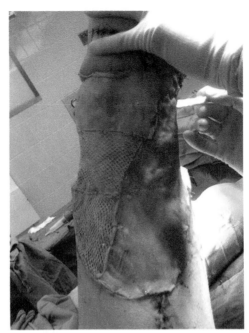

Fig. 4. Split thickness skin grafting of the site of controlled necrotizing skin and soft tissue infection.

should be applied in the first procedure, and a second look in the operating room should always be planned within 12 to 24 hours. Multiple looks in the operating room might be needed to ensure cessation of progression of the necrosis and infection. The wound should be closed or grafted only when all necrotic tissue has been debrided. When NSSTIs involve limbs, amputation might be indicated to control infection and prevent overwhelming septic shock. Fournier gangrene occasionally necessitates creation of a diverting ostomy to allow healing of the open wound without continuous fecal contamination. Early involvement of reconstructive surgeons is recommended, because many recovering patients are disfigured and will require complex flap closures and reconstructions (**Figs. 4** and **5**).

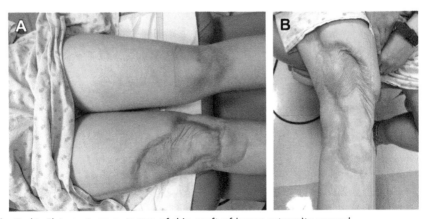

Fig. 5. (*A, B*) Long-term outcome of skin graft of lower extremity wound.

Table 2
The Infectious Diseases Society of America guidelines for antibiotic treatment of NSSTIs

First-line Antimicrobial Agent, by Infection Type	Adult Dosage	Antimicrobial Agents for Patients with Severe Penicillin Hypersensitivity
Mixed infection		
Ampicillin-sulbactam	1.5–3.0 g every 6–8 h iv	Clindamycin or metronidazole[a] with an amino-glycoside or fluoroquinolone
or		
Piperacillin-tazobactam	3.37 g every 6–8 h iv	
plus		
Clindamycin	600–900 mg/kg every 8 h iv	
plus		
Ciprofloxacin	400 mg every 12 h iv	
Imipenem/cilastatin	1 g every 6–8 h iv	—
Meropenem	1 g every 8 h iv	—
Ertapenem	1 g every day iv	—
Cefotaxime	2 g every 6 h iv	—
plus		
Metronidazole	500 mg every 6 h iv	
or		
Clindamycin	600–900 mg/kg every 8 h iv	
Streptococcus infection		
Penicillin	2–4 MU every 4–6 h iv (adults)	Vancomycin, linezolid, quinupristin/dalfopristin, or daptomycin
plus		
Clindasmycin	600–900 mg/kg every 8 h iv	
S aureus infection		
Nafcillin	1–2 g every 4 h iv	Vancomycin, linezolid, quinupristin/dalfopristin, daptomycin
Oxacillin	1–2 g every 4 h iv	—
Cefazolin	1 g every 8 h iv	—
Vancomycin (for resistant strains)	30 mg/kg/day in 2 divided doses iv	—
Clindamycin	600–900 mg/kg every 8 h iv	Bacteriostatic; potential of cross-resistance and emergence of resistance in erythromycin-resistant strains; inducible resistance in methicillin-resistant *S aureus*
Clostridium infection		
Clindamycin	600–900 mg/kg every 8 h iv	—
Penicillin	2–4 MU every 4–6 h iv	—

[a] If *Staphylococcus* infection is present or suspected, add an appropriate agent.

Broad Spectrum Antibiotics

As soon as an NSSTI is suspected, broad-spectrum antibiotics should be instituted. The optimal antibiotic regimen is controversial, but, as a rule, the regimen should address gram-positive, gram-negative, and anaerobic bacteria. A combination of a carbapenem (eg, imipenem, meropenem, ertapenem) or a β-lactam/β-lactamase inhibitor (eg, piperacillin/tazobactam) or cephalosporin (eg, cefepime) with an anti-methicillin-resistant*Staphylococcus aureus* agent (eg, vancomycin, linezolid) and an anti-anaerobic agent (eg, metronidazole or clindamycin) is a reasonable starting empiric regimen.[7] Clindamycin has additional antitoxin activity in addition to its anti-bacterial effects. Antibiotic coverage should be narrowed down as soon as Gram stain and culture results are available. The Infectious Diseases Society of America guidelines for NSSTIs are reported in **Table 2**.[8]

Hyperbaric Oxygen

The utility of hyperbaric oxygen in the treatment of NSSTI is controversial. There is hardly any level 1 data supporting its use, although multiple small retrospective studies reported decreased mortality with hyperbaric therapy.[9,10] In the authors' opinion, the logistic difficulties associated with transferring a critically ill patient to a hyperbaric chamber and providing nursing care to that patient in a hyperbaric chamber might outweigh the potential benefit the patient gets from the hyperbaric oxygen treatment.

Immunoglobulins

Intravenous immunoglobulins can neutralize the exotoxins secreted by clostridia and might also be effective against streptococcal superantigens. There are limited data suggesting a survival benefit of intravenous immunoglobulins in critically ill patients with group A streptococci NSSTIs, but the data are small and nondefinitive.[11–13]

PROGNOSIS

NSSTIs are associated with an elevated mortality (14%–50%). Factors associated with higher mortality include age greater than 60 years, heart disease, liver cirrhosis, leukocytosis greater than 30,000/mL, creatinine greater than 2.0 mg/dL, partial thmoboplastin time greater than 60 seconds, bandemia greater than 10%, bacteremia, soft tissue air on radiological imaging, and aeromonas or clostridial infection.[14,15] Delaying operative debridement has also been suggested as an independent predictor of mortality, again emphasizing the necessity of early and aggressive surgical intervention once the diagnosis has been suspected or confirmed.[16,17]

REFERENCES

1. O'Loughlin RE, Roberson A, Cieslak PR, et al. The epidemiology of invasive group A streptococcal infection and potential vaccine implications: United States, 2000-2004. Clin Infect Dis 2007;45(7):853–62.
2. Quirk WF Jr, Sternbach G. Joseph Jones: infection with flesh eating bacteria. J Emerg Med 1996;14(6):747–53.
3. Wong CH, Khin LW, Heng KS, et al. The LRINEC Laboratory (Risk Indicator for Necrotizing Fasciitis) score: a tool for distinguishing necrotizing fasciitis from other soft tissue infections. Crit Care Med 2004;32(7):1535–41.
4. Wilson MP, Schneir AB. A case of necrotizing fasciitis with a LRINEC score of zero: clinical suspicion should trump scoring systems. J Emerg Med 2013; 44(5):928–31.
5. Holland MJ. Application of the laboratory risk indicator in necrotising fasciitis (LRINEC) score to patients in a tropical tertiary referral centre. Anaesth Intensive Care 2009;37(4):588–92.

6. Dellinger RP, Levy MM, Rhodes A, et al. Surviving sepsis campaign: international guidelines for management of severe sepsis and septic shock, 2012. Intensive Care Med 2013;39(2):165–228.
7. Weigelt J, Itani K, Stevens D, et al, Linezolid CSSTI Study Group. Linezolid versus vancomycin in treatment of complicated skin and soft tissue infections. Antimicrob Agents Chemother 2005;49(6):2260–6.
8. Stevens DL, Bisno AL, Chambers HF, et al, Infectious Diseases Society of America. Practice guidelines for the diagnosis and management of skin and soft-tissue infections. Clin Infect Dis 2005;41(10):1373–406.
9. Brown DR, Davis NL, Lepawsky M, et al. A multicenter review of the treatment of major truncal necrotizing infections with and without hyperbaric oxygen therapy. Am J Surg 1994;167(5):485–9.
10. Hollabaugh RS Jr, Dmochowski RR, Hickerson WL, et al. Fournier's gangrene: therapeutic impact of hyperbaric oxygen. Plast Reconstr Surg 1998;101(1): 94–100.
11. Kaul R, McGeer A, Norrby-Teglund A, et al. Intravenous immunoglobulin therapy for streptococcal toxic shock syndrome—a comparative observational study. The Canadian Streptococcal Study Group. Clin Infect Dis 1999;28(4):800–7.
12. Norrby-Teglund A, Muller MP, Mcgeer A, et al. Successful management of severe group A streptococcal soft tissue infections using an aggressive medical regimen including intravenous polyspecific immunoglobulin together with a conservative surgical approach. Scand J Infect Dis 2005;37(3):166–72.
13. Darenberg J, Ihendyane N, Sjölin J, et al. Intravenous immunoglobulin G therapy in streptococcal toxic shock syndrome: a European randomized, double-blind, placebo-controlled trial. Clin Infect Dis 2003;37(3):333–40.
14. Huang KF, Hung MH, Lin YS, et al. Independent predictors of mortality for necrotizing fasciitis: a retrospective analysis in a single institution. J Trauma 2011;71(2): 467–73.
15. Anaya DA, McMahon K, Nathens AB, et al. Predictors of mortality and limb loss in necrotizing soft tissue infections. Arch Surg 2005;140(2):151–7.
16. Wong CH, Chang HC, Pasupathy S, et al. Necrotizing fasciitis: clinical presentation, microbiology, and determinants of mortality. J Bone Joint Surg Am 2003; 85-A(8):1454–60.
17. Childers BJ, Potyondy LD, Nachreiner R, et al. Necrotizing fasciitis: a fourteen-year retrospective study of 163 consecutive patients. Am Surg 2002;68(2): 109–16.

Acute Mesenteric Ischemia

Michael J. Sise, MD[a,b],*

KEYWORDS

- Acute mesenteric ischemia • Mesenteric arterial occlusion
- Mesenteric venous thrombosis • Nonocclusive mesenteric ischemia
- Ischemic colitis

KEY POINTS

- Acute mesenteric ischemia is uncommon and always occurs in the setting of preexisting comorbidities. Consequently mortality rates remain high.
- The 4 major types of acute mesenteric ischemia are acute superior mesenteric artery (SMA) thromboembolic occlusion, mesenteric arterial thrombosis, mesenteric venous thrombosis, and nonocclusive mesenteric ischemia, including ischemic colitis.
- Delays in diagnosis are common and associated with a high rate of morbidity and mortality.
- Prompt diagnosis requires attention to the history and physical examination, a high index of suspicion, and early contract CT scanning.
- Although both open and endovascular techniques have a role, operative management with exploratory laparotomy to asses bowel viability remains the best tool to prevent bowel infarction and an associated high mortality rate.
- Selective use of nonoperative therapy with volume resuscitation, optimizing cardiac output, and vasodilators has an important role in nonocclusive mesenteric ischemia of both the small bowel and colon.

OVERVIEW

Acute mesenteric ischemia remains a deadly process despite more than 50 years of advances in the treatment of vascular diseases. Successful management requires early diagnosis and prompt treatment if there is any chance of survival. The mortality rate remains more than 50% and there is little room for either delay or errors in management of this acute care surgical emergency.[1–4] Mesenteric ischemia is always secondary to a preexisting local or remote disease process and the cause ranges from cardiac source embolism to thrombosis of mesenteric veins in the setting of inherited or acquired hypercoagulability (**Box 1**).[3–5] Each type of mesenteric ischemia creates a

[a] Department of Surgery, University of California San Diego School of Medicine, San Diego, CA, USA; [b] Division of Trauma, Scripps Mercy Hospital, 4077 5th Avenue MER-62, San Diego, CA 92103, USA
* 550 Washington Street, Suite 641, San Diego, CA 92103.
E-mail address: Sise.mike@scrippshealth.org

Surg Clin N Am 94 (2014) 165–181
http://dx.doi.org/10.1016/j.suc.2013.10.012
0039-6109/14/$ – see front matter © 2014 Elsevier Inc. All rights reserved.

> **Box 1**
> **Associated diseases leading to mesenteric ischemia**
>
> *Mesenteric arterial occlusion*
> - Cardiac disease
>   - Atrial fibrillation
>   - Recent myocardial infarction
>   - Congestive heart failure
>   - Digitalis therapy
> - Previous arterial emboli
> - Hypercoagulable state
> - Hypovolemia, shock
>
> *Venous thrombosis*
> - Portal hypertension
> - Intra-abdominal inflammation
> - Trauma or major bowel surgery
> - Hypercoagulable state
> - Chronic renal failure

high risk of mesenteric infarction and death if diagnosis and treatment are delayed. Symptoms may vary from the sudden onset of diffuse, severe, and constant abdominal pain to the insidious onset of vague generalized abdominal pain. There are 4 common causes: acute cardiac source embolism to the SMA, acute thrombosis of preexisting stenotic atherosclerotic lesion, splanchnic vasoconstriction leading to low flow and regional ischemia (commonly called nonocclusive mesenteric ischemia) in either small or large bowel, and mesenteric venous thrombosis (**Table 1**).[6]

The purpose of this article is to review the pathophysiology, clinical presentation, diagnostic work-up, effective management, and outcome of acute mesenteric ischemia. Readers should acquire an increased sense of awareness of mesenteric ischemia, develop an appropriately high index of suspicion in a variety of clinical settings, and be ready to move with decisive action to promptly make the diagnosis and effectively manage it in a timely fashion.

MESENTERIC VASCULAR ANATOMY AND PHYSIOLOGY

The celiac artery and SMA origins from the aorta are in close proximity to the renal artery origins in the upper abdomen (**Fig. 1**). The celiac axis lies just below the aortic hiatus of the diaphragm. The proximal portions of the celiac artery and SMA are each enveloped

Table 1 Causes of mesenteric ischemia	
50%	Arterial embolism
20%	Arterial thrombosis
20%	Small vessel occlusion
10%	Venous thrombosis

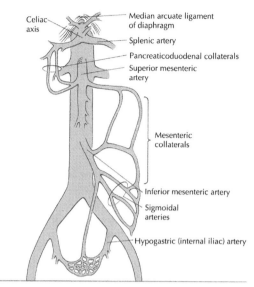

Celiac axis
Median arcuate ligament of diaphragm
Splenic artery
Pancreaticoduodenal collaterals
Superior mesenteric artery
Mesenteric collaterals
Inferior mesenteric artery
Sigmoidal arteries
Hypogastric (internal iliac) artery

Fig. 1. Mesenteric arterial anatomy demonstrating collateral flow between major branches of the aorta. (*From* Creager MA. Atlas of Vascular Disease. 2nd Edition. Philadelphia: Current Medicine 2003; with kind permission of Springer Science+Business Media.)

in a plexus of lymphatic and neurologic tissue. These vessels are relatively thin walled compared with extremity arteries. The portal vein and major mesenteric veins are also thin walled. The inferior mesenteric artery (IMA) arises from the left anterior lateral aspect of the mid-infrarenal aorta. The arterial blood supply of the gut is divided into 4 major areas (**Table 2**). Anomalous patterns of mesenteric arterial anatomy occur in approximately 15% of individuals and, although a replaced right hepatic artery from the SMA is one of the most commonly reported, there are a variety of anomalies reported.[6,7]

Table 2
Gut regions, arterial blood supply, and sources of collateral flow

Region	Blood Supply	Collateral Connections
Foregut: distal esophagus through the ampulla of Vater in the duodenum	Celiac artery	Pancreaticoduodenal arteries and arc of Bühler distally <5%
Migut: ampulla of Vater region of the duodenum to splenic flexure of the colon	SMA	Pancreaticoduodenal arteries and arc of Bühler proximally Marginal artery of Drummond and arc of Riolan distally
Hindgut: splenic flexure of the colon to distal sigmoid colon	IMA	Proximal: marginal artery of Drummond Distal: superior hemorrhoidal to middle hemorrhoidal arteries arc of Riolan
Cloacal derivatives: distal sigmoid colon, rectum colon, and anus	Branches of the internal iliac arteries	Middle hemorrhoidal to superior hemorrhoidal arteries proximally

Each of the mesenteric vessels interconnects with adjacent areas via preexisting collaterals. These collaterals have varying capability of supplying adequate blood supply to adjacent areas in acute occlusion. The gastroduodenal artery branch of the common hepatic artery anastomoses with branches of the inferior pancreatic duodenal artery. The dorsal pancreatic artery, a branch of the splenic artery, anastomoses with the anterior and posterior pancreaticoduodenal arcades via a right transverse branch of the dorsal pancreatic artery (Kirk's arcade). The arc of Bühler, which is present in only 1% to 4% of individuals, parallels the aorta proximally connecting the celiac axis to the SMA.[6] There may also be arcs of Barkow, collateral pathway within the omentum between the epiploic arteries of the splenic artery and SMA.[6]

In chronic atherosclerotic disease, the celiac axis distribution of flow may be adequately perfused from the SMA via the collaterals (described previously). They may also provide reverse flow to collateralize the SMA in chronic stenosis of its origin. These connections are usually inadequate, however, in acute SMA occlusion. The mesenteric arcades and the marginal artery of Drummond may provide adequate flow from the SMA to the IMA in the setting of occlusion at its origin. An important collateral, the arc of Riolan, develops in chronic occlusive disease and may provide flow in either direction between the proximal SMA and IMA. If the proximal IMA is occluded, the hypogastric arteries usually provide adequate collateral flow to the IMA distribution via the superior hemorrhoidal artery. The arc of Riolan is also an important collateral via the IMA to the hypogastric and iliac arteries to supply the lower extremities in chronic atherosclerotic infrarenal aortic occlusion.

In chronic mesenteric occlusive disease from atherosclerosis, patients may have total gut perfusion via a single remaining mesenteric artery or the bilateral hypogastric arteries via collateral flow to the other vessels.[7] Many of these patients, however, have intestinal angina when eating large meals.

The pattern of occlusion also determines if collaterals are adequate (**Fig. 2**). Emboli to the SMA usually lodge distal to the proximal jejunal branches and middle colic artery, thereby preventing celiac artery and IMA collateral contributions from reaching the small bowel and right colon.[6,8] Thrombotic occlusion of an atherosclerotic plaque at the origin of any of the mesenteric vessels often leaves collateral flow intact so that symptoms may not occur at bowel rest. If thrombosis extends distally in the SMA, however, a pattern of ischemia similar to acute embolism may occur.[7]

Venous drainage of the bowel is via the portal venous system (**Fig. 3**).[8] Gastric venous drainage is via the splenic vein and small bowel and the proximal colon through the splenic flexure drain via the superior mesenteric vein. The inferior mesenteric vein drains the descending colon and rectum. Collateral venous vessels are present between each major area of the portal venous drainage. Connection to the systemic venous system, however, is limited. Collateral flow via portal-systemic anastomoses in the area of the distal esophagus, the falciform ligament, and the anorectal area are well developed in chronic portal venous hypertension from hepatic parenchymal disease or chronic hepatic vein obstruction. They do not, however, provide adequate flow in acute total obstruction from portal vein thrombosis.[8]

Total mesenteric blood flow represents approximately 20% (varying between 10% and 35%) of resting cardiac output.[9] Postprandial blood flow may increase by as much as 200%. Symptoms, therefore, may relate to eating in patients with marginal collateral flow and acute occlusion.[10,11] The splanchnic circulation is also sensitive to the systemic effects of dehydration, inflammation, catecholamine release, cardiac insufficiency, and vigorous exercise. Each of these factors may result in nonocclusive mesenteric ischemia secondary to splanchnic vasoconstriction. In the setting of

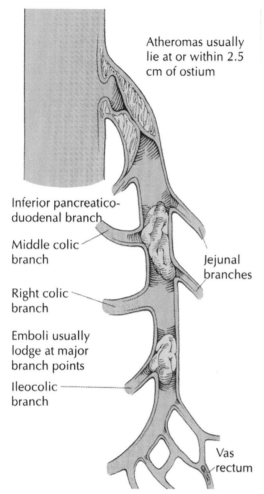

Atheromas usually lie at or within 2.5 cm of ostium

Inferior pancreatico-duodenal branch

Middle colic branch

Jejunal branches

Right colic branch

Emboli usually lodge at major branch points

Ileocolic branch

Vas rectum

Fig. 2. Location of proximal atherosclerotic thrombosis versus embolic occlusion in the SMA. (*From* Creager MA. Atlas of Vascular Disease. 2nd Edition. Philadelphia: Current Medicine 2003; with kind permission of Springer Science+Business Media.)

chronic atherosclerotic occlusive disease of the mesenteric vessels, these factors may precipitate mesenteric infarction from low flow.[9]

PATHOPHYSIOLOGY

The pathophysiology of mesenteric ischemia is essentially the result of insufficient blood flow to meet the metabolic demand of the bowel.[10,11] Acute ischemia leads to anaerobic metabolism in the gut, regional acidosis, and initial hyperperistalsis with cramping pain and gut emptying, followed by intense ischemic pain from gut wall hypoperfusion. This visceral pain is vague and projected across the area of the superficial abdominal wall where its innervation is shared with the surface structure innervation.[12] Therefore, foregut structures generate visceral pain in the epigastrium, midgut in the periumbilical regions, hindgut in the infrabumbilical region, and cloacal derivatives in the suprapubic region of the abdomen.[12]

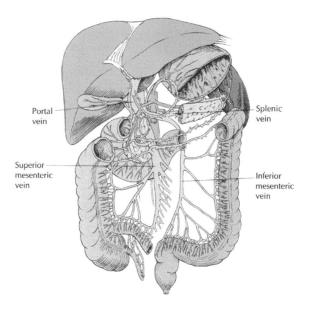

Portal vein

Splenic vein

Superior mesenteric vein

Inferior mesenteric vein

Fig. 3. Mesenteric and portal venous anatomy. (*From* Creager MA. Atlas of Vascular Disease. 2nd Edition. Philadelphia: Current Medicine 2003; with kind permission of Springer Science+Business Media.)

The bowel can tolerate marked reductions in blood flow.[9] At bowel rest, up to 80% of capillaries are not perfused without compromising adequate oxygen delivery. The intestinal mucosa extracts increasing amounts of oxygen during hypoperfusion and preserves mucosal integrity during initial periods of ischemia. Prolonged ischemia produces an inflammatory reaction, which disrupts the intestinal mucosal barrier and ultimately allows translocation of bacteria. Local peritoneal and systemic inflammatory sequelae follow quickly once transmural necrosis has occurred.[13]

Ischemia visceral pain is intense and constant, does not increase with palpation, and is not associated with abdominal wall rigidity or peritoneal signs on physical examination during its initial phases.[12] This results in the classic "pain out of proportion to physical findings" attributed to acute mesenteric ischemia. The initial gut emptying with vomiting may confuse an examining physician and divert attention to other gastrointestinal diagnoses. In the later stages with peritoneal inflammation, localization of pain in the abdomen and the presence of associated physical findings occur.

Cardiac source emboli have a predilection to enter the orifice of SMA most likely because of both its size and angle of origin from the aorta. SMA emboli typically lodge distal to the origin of proximal jejunal branches and the middle colic artery (see **Fig. 2**).[7] This gives rise to a pattern of small intestine and colon ischemia with sparing of the proximal jejunum and perfusion of the transverse colon and distal colon. Celiac artery and IMA emboli are less common and hypogastric artery emboli rarely cause ischemia due to the extent of pelvic collateral arteries.[7] Acute thrombosis of chronic atherosclerotic mesenteric arterial occlusive disease may result in a spectrum of symptoms from vague pain worsened by meals to sudden and intense pain identical to that of acute embolic occlusion. These symptoms depend on the preexisting collateral flow.

Mesenteric venous thrombosis is usually partially occlusive in its initial stages and causes symptoms with eating, including vague abdominal pain and nausea.[14,15] Acute total occlusion of the portal vein causes abdominal pain similar to acute SMA occlusion in addition to producing abdominal distension and diffuse tenderness due to intestinal venous engorgement and fluid sequestration in the abdomen. The late stages of intestinal ischemic syndromes are the result of intestinal infarction and systemic inflammatory response. Cardiovascular collapse may result if resection of necrotic bowel is not promptly performed. Mortality rates are prohibitively high with intestinal infarction.

Colon ischemia, usually resulting from either chronic mesenteric arterial insufficiency or nonocclusive mesenteric ischemia, is most common in the descending and sigmoid colon.[16,17] Regional hypoperfusion results in a spectrum of sequelae from mucosal sloughing to transmural infarction. The spectrum of symptoms often mimics diverticular disease. Bleeding, local inflammation, perforation with peritonitis, and late stricture may occur depending on the extent, severity, and duration of the ischemia. Transverse colon and right colon involvement may also occur in nonocclusive mesenteric ischemia.

CLINICAL PRESENTATION AND DIAGNOSIS

Acute intestinal ischemia from sudden embolic occlusion of the SMA causes the classic findings (described previously). Acute superimposed on chronic occlusion of a preexisting atherosclerotic disease often results in a more insidious onset of pain due to preexisting collateral flow, which mitigates the severity of ischemia.[10,11,18] A history of intestinal angina (postprandial pain), fear of food, and weight loss often accompanies acute on chronic mesenteric occlusive ischemia. Mesenteric venous thrombosis causes an insidious onset of initially vague symptoms, which worsen progressively over time.[14,15] In patients with inherited hypercoagulability, it may occur spontaneously or after a brief episode of gastreoenteritis or other illness. Mesenteric venous thrombosis from acquired hypercoagulability may occur in the conjunction with abdominal or multisystem trauma, intra-abdominal inflammation, or oral contraceptives. The most common causes are listed in **Box 1**.[14,15] Nonocclusive acute mesenteric ischemia from vasoconstriction occurs in the setting of critical illness with reduced cardiac output with or without preexisting mesenteric arterial stenosis. It is particularly difficult to diagnose in the critical care setting because it is associated with vague symptoms or undetectable symptoms in an intubated patient.

Atrial fibrillation is the most common cause of cardiac source embolism.[10,11,18] These patients describe a sudden onset of pain associated with nausea, vomiting, and diarrhea. The most common initial findings are mild abdominal distension and hypoactive bowel sounds without abdominal tenderness. In patients with acute worsening of chronic mesenteric ischemia, almost all have a history of postprandial pain and weight loss (**Table 3**).

Profound leukocytosis may be the only initial abnormal laboratory studies in patients with acute mesenteric ischemia and the white blood cell counts often exceed 20,000 cmm.[10,18] All patients with abdominal pain and a profound leukocytosis should have intestinal ischemia included in their differential diagnoses. Metabolic acidosis is a

Table 3	
Frequency of signs and symptoms in chronic mesenteric arterial occlusive disease	
1. Postprandial pain	100%
2. Weight loss	85%
3. Abdominal bruit	70%
4. Nausea, vomiting	60%

late finding and indicates intestinal infarction. Because of the liver's ability to clear lactic acid, however, the early stages of intestinal infarction do not result in systemic metabolic acidosis. Hyperamylasemia and elevated serum lipase may also occur in the early course of mesenteric ischemia.[1,2,10,19]

An early diagnosis of acute mesenteric ischemia in patients at risk requires a promptly performed CT scan of the abdomen with intravenous contrast.[20,21] This examination effectively evaluates mesenteric arterial and venous patency and perfusion of the bowel and indicates if one of the other possible causes of clinical findings is present. Early CT scanning both allows timely diagnosis before significant bowel compromise occurs and makes appropriate interventions more likely to succeed.[1,2,20,21] Intestinal necrosis may cause an overwhelming inflammatory response and shock with an associated high mortality rate.[13,22] One of the primary reasons why the outcome of acute mesenteric ischemia has not significantly improved in the past 4 decades is the all too common delay in diagnosis and intestinal infarction in this group of patients who are all at risk because of the high incidence of significant comorbidities.[12,22–24] The best strategy to improve outcomes remains prompt recognition, early diagnosis, and successful management prior to bowel necrosis.[1,2,12]

The role of catheter angiography of the mesenteric vessels has diminished with the availability of CT angiography. The timesavings with immediately available CT imaging and the morbidity of catheterization both make this traditional diagnostic technique unnecessary. Endovascular techniques have a role, however, in managing mesenteric ischemia (discussed later). The widespread use of CT imaging has resulted in improved early diagnosis and an improvement in outcomes.

MANAGEMENT OF MESENTERIC ISCHEMIA

The key principles of management of acute mesenteric ischemia are summarized in **Fig. 4**. The decision for an immediate open surgical approach versus an endovascular approach requires consideration of 3 key factors. First and foremost is the duration and severity of bowel ischemic, followed by the nature of the occlusive lesion, and equally important is consideration of the ready availability and the capability of an

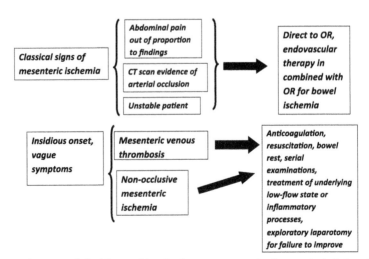

Fig. 4. Key elements of decision making in the management of mesenteric ischemia.

emergency center's interventional radiology or vascular surgical intervention program.[1,2,10,25] In patients with suspected bowel infarction or impending infarction, immediate exploratory laparotomy is mandatory.[2,25] At exploration, the cause of mesenteric ischemia is found and remedied and bowel viability is assessed. Embolic occlusion usually is due to a relatively organized cardiac thrombus, which is not amenable to thrombolytic therapy. Thrombolysis also risks fragmentation and further distal embolization, which cannot be further lysed or retrieved by catheter thrombectomy. Bowel infarction is likely to result. Therefore, prompt operation with SMA embolectomy combined with inspection of the bowel for necrosis is the best approach. The operative technical aspects of the management of each major cause of acute mesenteric ischemia are summarized in **Fig. 5**.

Acute thrombosis of chronic atherosclerotic occlusive disease may be managed with endovascular techniques, with stenting the mesenteric arterial lesion.[10,11,26–29] Thrombolytic therapy has a role in the treatment of fresh thrombus in this cause of acute mesenteric ischemia.[10,11,28,29] Successful use of these endovascular techniques requires, however, an active preexisting program with adequate personnel, equipment, and timely staffing at the emergency center. Even if thrombolysis and stenting are successful, exploratory laparotomy may be required to assess the recovery of ischemic bowel. The risk of bowel necrosis and subsequent peritonitis requires prompt abdominal exploration in those patients who do not have complete relief of symptoms and the absence of signs of ongoing ischemia after endovascular techniques. Laparoscopy has a limited role in the management of mesenteric ischemia.[10,11,25]

Intraoperative assessment of intestinal blood flow includes running the bowel and inspection of the entire intestinal tract by assessing color and peristaltic activity and palpating the mesenteric arterial arcades. The main trunk of the SMA is located by upward retraction the transverse colon and downward retraction of the small bowel. The trunk of the artery is palpated at the root of the mesentery along the inferior margin of the body of the pancreas. The celiac artery and its branches are palpated through the lesser sac in the midline over the aorta just below the left lobe of the liver. The IMA is

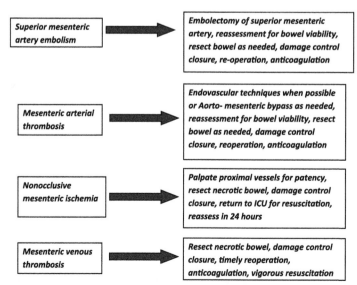

Fig. 5. Summary of intraoperative management of acute mesenteric ischemia.

located by inspection along left anterior-lateral area of the infrarenal aorta at the base of the left colon mesentery. Assessment of the distal mesenteric at the bowel for Doppler signals aids in the assessment of areas of questionable perfusion. Fluorescein angiography with an ultraviolet lamp can be helpful in further assessing the return of perfusion.[30]

If mesenteric ischemia is first encountered in the operating room, the pattern and appearance of ischemic bowel are essential in determining the cause (**Fig. 6**).[1,10,11] Embolism to the SMA usually lodges in the main trunk of the vessel distal to the origin of the proximal jejunal branches and the middle colic artery. This results in proximal sparing of the jejunum and distal sparing of the transverse colon with ischemia of the remaining small bowel and ascending colon. Thrombosis of the SMA origin leads to ischemia throughout its distribution from the duodenum to the splenic flexure of the

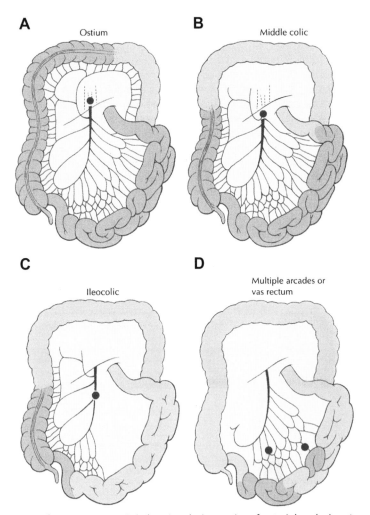

Fig. 6. Patterns of acute mesenteric ischemia relative to site of arterial occlusion. Location of SMA occlusion (*A*) Ostium, (*B*) Below middle colic artery, (*C*) At ileocolic vessels, (*D*) Multiple arcades or vas rectum. (*From* Creager MA. Atlas of Vascular Disease. 2nd Edition. Philadelphia: Current Medicine 2003; with kind permission of Springer Science+Business Media.)

colon. Total visceral ischemia from the distal esophagus through the rectum results if the celiac artery and the IMA are also occluded. This rare phenomenon may present with a hungry and hypoglycemic patient secondary to the loss of liver perfusion and access to glycogen stores and carries a poor prognosis.

EMBOLIC MESENTERIC ARTERIAL OCCLUSION

SMA emboli are best removed through a transverse incision in the main trunk of the artery at the mesenteric root below the pancreas (**Fig. 7**).[11,31] Fogarty catheter embolectomy must be performed with caution (**Fig. 8**). This visceral artery is fragile and catheters should be used gently proximally and distally to avoid arterial injury from tears and dissections. Once thrombectomy is completed, careful flushing with heparinized saline (10 units of heparin per mL) proximally and distally is performed. Avoid flushing forcibly proximally to prevent dislodging thrombus into the aorta and causing distal embolism. Closure of the arteriotomy should be performed in a tension-free manner with either running or interrupted monofilament sutures by placing proximal and distal vascular clamps and gently retracting the artery toward the arterotomy site. After re-establishing flow, placing warm laparotomy packs and waiting 10 to 15 minutes to reassess are helpful in relieving spasm. Damage control closure and reinspection in 24 to 36 hours is advised unless there is prompt complete restoration of normal intestinal blood flow without questionable areas of bowel at the initial operation.[10,11]

THROMBOTIC MESENTERIC ARTERIAL OCCLUSION

Proximal mesenteric arterial thrombosis and acute bowel ischemia discovered in the operating room require experience in advanced vascular surgical technique.[10,11,26] If an acute care surgeon is not comfortable and capable of performing the necessary aortomesenteric bypass, a vascular surgeon colleague should be called for assistance. There are a variety of bypass options. Retrograde iliac artery to mesenteric artery bypass is seemingly easier to perform than antegrade supraceliac arotomesenteric bypass. Retrograde bypasses may, however, yield inferior results.[32–35] In

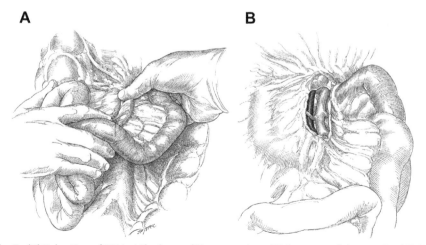

Fig. 7. (*A*) Palpation of SMA at the base of the mesentery. (*B*) Exposure of the proximal SMA. (*From* Rutherford RB. Atlas of Vascular Surgery. Philadelphia, W.B. Saunders 1993; with permission.)

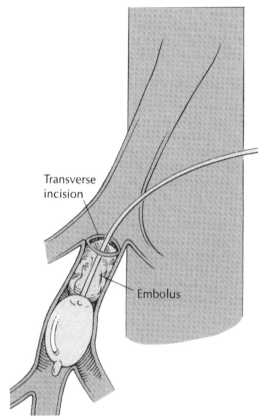

Fig. 8. Balloon catheter embolectomy of the SMA. (*From* Creager MA. Atlas of Vascular Disease. 2nd Edition. Philadelphia: Current Medicine 2003; with kind permission of Springer Science+Business Media.)

patients with proximal mesenteric atherosclerotic occlusive disease, the iliac arteries are usually also involved. It may be difficult to find a suitable graft origin site in the iliac arteries and it is also difficult to complete without kinking. This bypass route also places synthetic graft in proximity to the duodenum, and eventual and graft erosion and graft infection or graft-enteric fistula are risks.

Antegrade aortomesenteric bypass from the supraceliac aorta is the best choice for restoring flow in acute mesenteric ischemia from proximal mesenteric arterial thrombosis (**Fig. 9**).[32] This bypass should be performed by experienced surgeons and requires exposure of the retrocrural aorta by mobilizing the left lobe of the liver. The lesser omenetum is incised and the left hepatic lobe is retracted medially with the stomach retracted caudally. The aorta is palpated through the crura of the diaphragm and its fibers divided longitudinally to expose the area for the proximal end-to-side anastomosis to the aorta. Bypass to the SMA is performed by tunneling the graft with blunt dissection along the left anterior lateral aspect of the aorta behind the pancreas to the artery at the root of the mesentery. More proximal exposure of the SMA is achieved by direct dissection down the SMA behind the pancreas. There is dense plexus of lymphatic and neural tissue at the proximal SMA, which must be dissected free to expose as sufficient length of artery for distal anastomosis. If needed, the celiac artery origin is exposed in a similar fashion to its bifurcation into the splenic

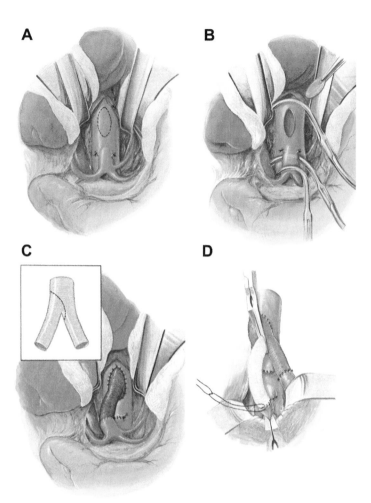

Fig. 9. Antegrade aortomesenteric artery bypass. (*A*) Exposure aorta behind crura of the diaphragm, (*B*) Create aortic site for anastomosis, (*C*) Graft for single vessel bypass, (*D*) Graft for bypass to both celiac artery and superior mesenteric artery. (*From* Wylie EJ, Stoney RJ, Ehrenfeld WK. Manual of Vascular Surgery Vol.1. New York: Springer-Verlag 1980; with kind permission of Springer Science+Business Media.)

and common hepatic branches in order to place a second bypass limb. Patients should be systemically heparinized (5000 units of heparin intravenous bolus) prior to arterial clamping the aorta. Proximal and distal totally occluding aortic clamps are preferred because partially occluding clamps may make anastomosis difficult and damage the aorta, causing dissection or distal emboli. The distal anastomoses should be performed in an end-to-side fashion with careful antegrade and retrograde flushing and, if indicated, balloon catheter thrombectomy. The bowel is then inspected for viability (described previously).

MESENTERIC VENOUS THROMBOSIS

The management of mesenteric ischemia from acute on chronic occlusive lesions should also include damage control techniques.[5,10,11,36] If there is any doubt regarding intestinal viability, damage control closure may be performed without increasing the risk of bypass infection. Necrotic bowel is best resected by stapling and dividing at healthy margins and anastamosis of bowel segments deferred until reoperation at 24 to 36 hours to make certain further necrosis and failure of the anastomosis do not occur. Expeditious temporary abdominal wall closure followed by prompt transfer to an ICU for further postoperative critical care management is crucial to manage these patients who are invariably hemodynamically unstable. Intravenous administration of heparin for anticoagulation hemorrhage to prevent rethrombosis of mesenteric vessels should occur early with damage control closures despite the risk of hemorrhage.

Mesenteric venous thrombosis leading to bowel necrosis is best treated nonoperatively with anticoagulation and adequate restoration of circulating blood volume.[14,15] Operative management is reserved for patients with sign of bowel infraction. Bowel resection of necrotic bowel segments is the only option in these advanced cases. Extensive resection is common when forced to operate and the prognosis is poor. Prompt recognition is frequently difficult because of the insidious onset of this form of deep venous thrombosis. It may be more difficult to manage than arterial source mesenteric ischemia.[14,15] By the time intestinal infarction occurs from venous engorgement and impeded arterial flow, there are few, if any, options that relieve venous congestion. The few mesenteric and portal venous thrombectomies reported have had poor results and this procedure is dangerous and not effective. Early recognition with systemic anticoagulation coupled with resection of necrotic bowel, damage control closure, and aggressive resuscitative measures are all essential for successful management of this often devastating type of mesenteric ischemia. Multiple reoperations to reassess bowel for viability are invariably required. Patients who survive often have undergone extensive bowel resection and are often left with short gut syndrome.[37]

NONOCCLUSIVE MESENTERIC ISCHEMIA

The setting of nonocclusive mesenteric ischemia, including ischemic colitis, almost always involves critical illness. Severe cardiopulmonary insufficiency and septic shock with the use of vasoconstricting drugs are the most common critical illnesses associated with this entity. The treatment is based on improving mesenteric perfusion and watchful waiting for the presence of bowel infarction. Optimizing volume status and limiting vasoconstriction by weaning vasopressor drug infusions are essential to improving mesenteric blood flow. The decision to perform exploratory laparotomy is based on the presence of signs of perforation or overall worsening status suggestive of bowel infarction.

At exploratory laparotomy for suspected bowel infarction, obvious areas of nonviable bowel must be expeditiously resected. Unless a patient is stable and the area of resection is adjacent to normal bowel on each margin, stapling across bowel, performing a damage control closure, and returning in 24 to 36 hours to reassess for the need for further resection are essential to successful management. This is particularly important when multiple areas of bowel resection are required.

Ischemic colitis is managed in a similar fashion to other areas of nonocclusive mesenteric ischemia. Bowel rest, antibiotics, and adequate fluid infusion lead to successful nonoperative management in more than 60% of patients. Signs of peritonitis or deteriorating hemodynamic status should prompt immediate exploratory laparotomy with appropriate bowel resection. Colostomy and a Hartmann procedure are often warranted.

OUTCOME

The frequently associated significant health problems and all too common delays in diagnosis have made acute mesenteric ischemia a highly morbid and often fatal disease process. The initial results are related to both the presence of intestinal infarction and the underlying causes of vascular compromise. Overall survival has not significantly changed in the past 4 decades. Perioperative mortality approaches 50%.[15,18,23,24,38–40] Recurrent cardiac source embolism occurs in 30% of patients with acute SMA embolism.[23,24] Mesenteric arterial thrombosis is a harbinger of systemic atherosclerosis and the risk of death from coronary artery disease is high. Mesenteric venous thrombosis is usually a secondary phenomenon and lifelong risk of thrombotic complications follows for those who survive.[3,14,15,37]

The most important factor in the care of patients with acute mesenteric ischemia is management of their underlying comorbidities. Some form of anticoagulation or antiplatelet therapy is required. Cardiac disease should be aggressively treated. The underlying causes of hypercoagulability must be delineated in those with mesenteric venous thrombosis. Lifelong medical management of their comorbidities is essential for all survivors of the various forms of mesenteric ischemia.

REFERENCES

1. Wyers MC. Acute mesenteric ischemia: diagnostic approach and surgical treatment. Semin Vasc Surg 2010;23:9–20.
2. Kougias P, Lau D, El Sayed FH, et al. Determinants of mortality and treatment outcome following surgical interventions for acute mesenteric ischemia. J Vasc Surg 2007;46:467–74.
3. Schoots IG, Koffeman GI, Legemate DA, et al. Systematic review of survival after acute mesenteric ischemia according to disease aetiology. Br J Surg 2004;91: 17–27.
4. Herbert GS, Steele SR. Acute and chronic mesenteric ischemia. Surg Clin North Am 2007;87:1115–34.
5. Schermerhorn ML, Giles KA, Hamdan AD, et al. Mesenteric revascularization: management and outcomes in the United States 1988–2006. J Vasc Surg 2009;50:341–8.
6. Walker TG. Mesenteric vasculature collateral pathways. Semin Intervent Radiol 2009;26:167–74.
7. Moore WS. Visceral ischemic syndromes. In: Moore WS, editor. Vascular and endovascular surgery. 7th edition. New York: Saunders; 2005.
8. Madhoff DC, de Baere T. Portal vein normal anatomy and variants: implication for liver surgery and portal vein embolization. Semin Intervent Radiol 2008;25:86–91.
9. Marston A, Clarke JM, Garcia Garcia J, et al. Intestinal function and intestinal blood supply: a 20 year surgical study. Gut 1985;26:656–66.
10. Oldenburg WA, Lau LL, Rodenberg TL, et al. Acute mesenteric ischemia. Arch Intern Med 2004;164:1054–62.
11. McKinsey JF, Gewertz BL. Acute mesenteric ischemia. Surg Clin North Am 1997; 77:307–18.
12. Curie DJ. Abdominal pain. London: Hemisphere Pub Corp; 1979.
13. Moore EE, Moore FA, Franciose RJ, et al. The postischemic gut serves as a priming bed for circulating neutrophils that provoke multiple organ failiure. J Trauma 1994;37:881–7.
14. Boley SJ, Kaleya RN, Brandt LJ. Mesenteric venous thrombosis. Surg Clin North Am 1992;72:183–201.

15. Rhee RY, Gloviczki P, Mendonca CT, et al. Mesenteric venous thrombosis: still a lethal disease in the 1990s. J Vasc Surg 1994;20:688–97.
16. Scharff JR, Longo WE, Vartanian SH, et al. Ischemic colitis: spectrum of disease and outcome. Surgery 2003;134:624–30.
17. Walker AM, Bohn RL, Cali C, et al. Risk factors for colon ischemia. Am J Gastroenterol 2004;99:1333–7.
18. Burns BJ, Brandt LJ. Intestinal ischemia. Gastroenterol Clin North Am 2003;32: 1127–43.
19. Horton KM, Fishman EK. Multidetector CT angiography in the diagnosis of mesenteric ischemia. Radiol Clin North Am 2007;45:275–88.
20. Cikrit DF, Harris VJ, Hemmer CG, et al. Comparison of spiral CT scan and arteriography for evaluation of renal and visceral arteries. Ann Vasc Surg 1996;10: 109–16.
21. Ridley N, Green SE. Mesenteric arterial thrombosis diagnosed on CT. Am J Roentgenol 2001;176:549.
22. Hassoun HT, Kone BC, Mercer DW, et al. Post-injury multiple organ failure: the role of the gut. Shock 2001;15:1–10.
23. Klempnauer J, Grothues F, Bekras H, et al. Long-term results after surgery for acute mesenteric ischemia. Surgery 1997;121:239–43.
24. Cho JS, Carr JA, Jacobsen G, et al. Long-term outcome after mesenteric artery reconstruction: a 37-year experience. J Vasc Surg 2002;35:453–60.
25. Endean ED, Barnes SL, Kwolek CJ, et al. Surgical Management of thrombotic acute intestinal ischemia. Ann Surg 2001;233:801–8.
26. Park WM, Gloviczki P, Cherry KJ, et al. Contemporary management of acute mesenteric ischemia: factors associated with survival. J Vasc Surg 2002;35: 445–52.
27. Hansen KJ, Wilson DB, Craven TE, et al. Mesenteric artery disease in the elderly. J Vasc Surg 2004;40:45–52.
28. Kasirajan K, O'Hara PJ, Gray BH, et al. Chronic mesenteric ischemia: open surgery versus percutaneous angioplasty and stenting. J Vasc Surg 2001;33:63–71.
29. Matsumoto AH, Angle JF, Spinosa DJ, et al. Percutaneous transluminal angioplasty and stenting in the treatment of chronic mesenteric ischemia: results and long-term follow up. J Am Coll Surg 2002;194:S22–31.
30. Ballard J, Stone W, Hallett J, et al. A critical analysis of adjuvant techniques used to assess bowel viability in acute mesenteric ischemia. Am Surg 1993;7:309–11.
31. Bjorek M, Acosta S, Lindber F, et al. Revascularization of the superior mesenteric artery after acute thromboembolic occlusion. Br J Surg 2002;89:923–7.
32. Hermeck J, Thomas JH, Ilipoulos JI, et al. Role of supraceliac aortic bypass in visceral artery reconstruction. Am J Surg 1991;162:611–4.
33. Foley MI, Moneta G, Abu-Zamzam AM, et al. Revascularization of the superior mesenteric artery alone for treatment of intestinal ischemia. J Vasc Surg 2000; 32:37–47.
34. Gentile A, Moneta G, Taylor L, et al. Isolated bypass to the superior mesenteric artery for intestinal ischemia. Arch Surg 1994;129:926–32.
35. Hirsch AT, Haskal ZJ, Hertzer NR, et al. ACC/AHA 2005 Practice guidelines for the management of patients with peripheral arterial disease (lower extremity, renal, mesenteric, and abdominal aortic). Circulation 2006;113:463–654.
36. Ryer EJ, Manju Kalra M, Oderich GS, et al. Revascularization for acute mesenteric ischemia. J Vasc Surg 2012;55:1682–9.
37. Thompson JS, Langnas AN, Pinch LW, et al. Surgical approach to short-bowel syndrome. Experience in a population of 160 patients. Ann Surg 1995;222:600–5.

38. Creager MA. Atlas of vascular disease. 2nd edition. Philadelphia: Current Medicine; 2003.
39. Rutherford RB. Atlas of vascular surgery. Philadelphia: W.B. Saunders; 1993.
40. Wylie EJ, Stoney RJ, Ehrenfeld WK. Manual of vascular surgery, vol. 1. New York: Springer-Verlag; 1980.

Thoracic Emergencies

Stephanie G. Worrell, MD, Steven R. DeMeester, MD*

KEYWORDS

- Upper airway obstruction • Massive hemoptysis • Spontaneous pneumothorax
- Pulmonary empyema

KEY POINTS

- Rigid bronchoscopy can handle almost any cause of airway obstruction.
- The current first-line treatment of managing massive hemoptysis is interventional radiology embolization after stabilization of the airway.
- The decision to surgically treat for prevention of recurrence depends on the cause and to some extent the risk associated with recurrence.

ACUTE UPPER AIRWAY OBSTRUCTION

Introduction

The incidence of death from acute airway obstruction in adults increases with age and peaks at 85 years old.[1] The most common cause is aspiration of a foreign body. This situation leads to sudden obstruction of an otherwise normal airway in most instances. Other causes include trauma, inflammation, tumors, and neurologic diseases. Apart from trauma, these other causes are usually chronic, but when they reach a critical point, they present as acute airway obstruction. The most common cause of chronic airway obstruction is tracheal stenosis related to prior intubation. This condition accounts for approximately 90% of cases.[2] Intubations as short as 24 hours can lead to tracheal stenosis.[3] Often, patients with chronic airway compromise are asymptomatic at rest but may note stridor or dyspnea on exertion.

Critical stenosis occurs when the diameter of the airway has decreased to 25% or less of the normal tracheal diameter. The normal diameter varies for individuals and is typically 15 to 25 mm. In general, critical stenosis occurs when the diameter of the trachea is less than 4 mm (**Fig. 1**).

Anatomy/Pathophysiology

Upper airway obstruction is defined as an obstruction of the airway at any location from the mouth to the carina. The narrowest portion of the upper airway is the larynx

Disclosures: None.
Department of Surgery, Keck School of Medicine, University of Southern California, 1510 San Pablo Street, Suite 514, Los Angeles, CA 90033, USA
* Corresponding author.
E-mail address: steven.demeester@med.usc.edu

Surg Clin N Am 94 (2014) 183–191
http://dx.doi.org/10.1016/j.suc.2013.10.013
0039-6109/14/$ – see front matter © 2014 Elsevier Inc. All rights reserved.

surgical.theclinics.com

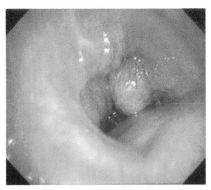 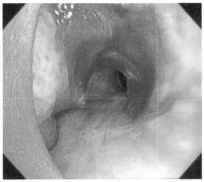

Fig. 1. Tracheal mass semiobstructing the airway before and after removal by coring out the mass.

at the glottis in adults and the subglottic region in infants. Most foreign body obstructions occur in this area. However, obstruction can occur at any location in the upper airway.

Clinical Presentation/Examination

Presenting signs and symptoms
Cough
Hoarseness
Shortness of breath
Dyspnea on exertion
Stridor (biphasic if within the extrathoracic trachea)
Use of accessory muscles
Nasal flaring
Chest wall retractions
Cyanosis
Decreased consciousness

Diagnosis

Rapid diagnosis and treatment are critical to patient survival. Complete upper airway obstruction can lead to cardiac arrest and death within minutes. Once stridor is present, the airway is already severely compromised. It is imperative to first assess the degree of obstruction. This situation can quickly be evaluated by the distress of the patient. Are they working hard to breathe? Can they talk?

The cause of upper airway obstruction can be broken down into 2 categories: aspiration versus nonaspiration. With aspiration, there is typically a clear history of the event. No endotracheal tube should be placed to avoid potentially pushing the object more distally in to the oropharynx. Instead, the Heimlich maneuver should be attempted if feasible. If this maneuver is not successful or feasible and the patient is stable and moving air, the safest option is to rapidly bring the patient to the operating room for a rigid bronchoscopy. If the patient has no airway or an inadequate airway, an immediate cricothyrotomy should be performed.

The second cause is nonaspiration, typically a stricture or tumor. If the patient is able to maintain a patent airway and time permits, a computed tomography (CT) scan should be obtained to define the level of obstruction. Again, no intubation should be attempted, because this may exacerbate the problem. After the CT scan, or immediately if the patient has an unstable airway, the patient should be taken to the operating room. While awaiting the operating room, heliox, a gaseous mixture of helium and oxygen, can be given to the patient. Heliox can temporize the airway and decrease the work of breathing before intervention. Initially, a flexible bronchoscopy can be performed, with minimal sedation if the patient is stable. This procedure allows an assessment of the cause and location of the obstruction. However, in most circumstances, the bronchoscope should not be advanced through the lesion, because even a small amount of blood or inflammation can convert a marginal airway into an emergent airway problem. In most circumstances, definitive management of a compromised airway is best performed with a rigid bronchoscope. These scopes allow coring out of an airway tumor and dilatation of a stricture, along with removal of secretions and any aspirated material. In some circumstances, balloon dilatation through a flexible bronchoscope is reasonable, but a rigid bronchoscope should be immediately available in case the balloon dilatation is unsuccessful or induces bleeding. Before beginning the procedure, it is imperative that everything is laid out so that all instruments are immediately accessible. The guiding principle is that once the procedure has begun, there is no time to find additional pieces of equipment or replacements without compromising the ability to save the patient. The light source should be attached to the rigid and the flexible bronchoscope and tested. In addition, a backup light source should be in the room. Useful adjuvant equipment includes the argon beam for hemostasis or further debridement of a tumor or stricture, and dilute epinephrine irrigation for hemostasis.

Once everything is assembled, a decision is made based on the status of the airway to initially evaluate with the flexible bronchoscope or to go in immediately with the rigid bronchoscope. When going in with a rigid bronchoscope, I prefer to rapidly paralyze the patient to avoid bucking and coughing, which can complicate an already high-risk procedure. However, once the patient is paralyzed, it is unlikely that mask respiration will be successful in someone with a compromised airway, so familiarity with rigid bronchoscopy is essential. Even when practitioners are very experienced, these situations are among the most stressful in all of medicine, because in most circumstances, there is little more than 2 minutes to establish an adequate airway.

Summary

Establishing an airway is the most critical component to treating a patient with upper airway obstruction. This is one of the most challenging and stressful situations in all of medicine. Often, there is only 2 to 3 minutes to save a patient's life and familiarity with rigid bronchoscopy is essential. Rigid bronchoscopy can handle almost any cause of airway obstruction.

MASSIVE HEMOPTYSIS
Introduction

Massive hemoptysis is usually defined as coughing up 600 mL or more of blood within 24 hours.[4] Mortality associated with massive hemoptysis ranges from 5% to 15%, mainly related to asphyxiation, as the airway fills with blood.[5–8] The main causes underlying massive hemoptysis include bronchiectasis, tuberculosis, mycetomas, necrotizing pneumonia, and bronchogenic carcinomas.[9] Patients with cystic fibrosis are also presenting at increasing rate and are at an increased risk of massive hemoptysis.[10]

The feeder vessels typically associated with massive hemoptysis include the bronchial, intercostal, and accessory arteries off the subclavian artery. Among the common causes (bronchiectasis, tuberculosis, and infection) the cause of bleeding is usually inflammation of the airway, with rupture of the bronchial arteries from dilation or ulceration. Rarely, the pulmonary artery can be associated with massive hemoptysis, as seen in Rasmussen aneurysm.

Clinical Presentation/Examination

Massive hemoptysis can be life threatening. The first steps when a patient presents are to establish a patent airway and volume resuscitate as necessary. After this stage, the most important step is to identify which lung is involved, right versus left, and then to establish which lobe is involved. To evaluate this situation, a chest radiograph and flexible bronchoscopy should be performed. A CT scan may be helpful to localize bleeding, but in general, angiography is preferred. Angiography is preferred because it can identify the source of bleeding and then treat with embolization in the same setting. Angiography has recently become the preferred first-line treatment. In patients with near airway obstruction from clotted blood, a rigid bronchoscopy may also be necessary. However, most patients can be managed with a flexible bronchoscope down a large endotracheal tube for suctioning of blood.

In general, intubation with a double lumen tube is avoided, because the small diameter of each lumen makes suctioning of the airway difficult. In cases of truly massive and continued hemoptysis, in which the side or lobe is known, a bronchial blocker or double lumen tube may temporize the situation until embolization or operative intervention is performed.

Technique

The airway should be suctioned with a bronchoscope to obtain a patent airway. Lavage with cold saline or vasoactive agents can be attempted; however, this is not so effective for massive hemoptysis. These techniques are more useful when used for postbiopsy-induced hemorrhage. This situation is in part because the agent is washed away by the brisk bleeding.[11] After stabilization of the airway, definitive treatment of the feeder vessel is required.

Interventional radiology (IR) with embolization is currently first-line therapy. There is a reported 10% to 29% recurrence rate, likely because of incomplete embolization, recanalization, or collateral circulation.[9] The following have been identified as risk factors for recurrent bleeding after IR embolization: residual mild bleeding beyond the first week after intervention, need for blood transfusion before the procedure, and aspergilloma as the cause for bleeding.[12] In these cases, IR embolization can be used as a temporizing measure while waiting for definitive surgical resection. There are some reports of successful medical treatment with oral and intravenous tranexamic acid in patients with cystic fibrosis who have failed multiple IR embolizations.[13] Failure of IR embolization may also indicate that the bronchial artery is not the source of the hemoptysis and that an additional feeder artery that has not been embolized may be the source. Repeated efforts to localize and embolize the source are reasonable options in a stable patient.

Surgery is being used less frequently, because of the high associated morbidity and mortality. Surgery remains the best option for patients with complex arteriovenous fistulas, iatrogenic pulmonary artery rupture, chest trauma, and recurrent life-threatening hemoptysis.[14] However, surgery is an option only if the source of bleeding has been localized to a side or lobe. With the addition of multimodality therapies, the morbidity and mortality associated with massive hemoptysis have dramatically improved.[4]

Summary

The current first-line treatment of managing massive hemoptysis is IR embolization after stabilization of the airway. It is important to localize the side and if possible the lobe that are the source of bleeding, with bronchoscopy and a chest radiograph. Surgical resection is reserved for bleeding that does not respond to embolization or in an unstable patient with ongoing massive hemoptysis in whom the lobe involved has been determined. The mortality with surgical resection, even in an elective setting, is high, particularly with upper lobe sources secondary to the dense inflammation usually associated with the underlying abnormality. Before any consideration of surgery, the side and preferably the lobe involved with the bleeding must be known. Once both lungs are filled with blood, it becomes difficult to identify the source, emphasizing the importance of early bronchoscopy to localize the side of bleeding.

SPONTANEOUS PNEUMOTHORAX
Introduction

Spontaneous pneumothorax (SP) is defined as air in the pleural space, which can occur as a primary or secondary cause. Primary SP occurs in patients with no known underlying lung disease. In these patients, a CT scan is not necessary. These patients are typically tall, thin men with low body mass index.[15–17] Secondary SP is associated with an underlying lung pathology, most commonly chronic obstructive pulmonary disease, cystic fibrosis, tuberculosis, and lung cancer. In these patients, a CT scan is useful to evaluate the underlying lung parenchyma.

Relevant Anatomy/Pathophysiology

A pneumothorax occurs when air collects between the visceral and parietal pleura. Air usually enters the pleural cavity though a ruptured bleb in the lung during inspiration and acts like a valve mechanism, allowing air to enter the pleural cavity, which cannot escape. Corresponding to the increase in pleural pressure, the ipsilateral lung collapses. This situation can progress to a tension pneumothorax if increased pressures cause the mediastinum to shift and impair the ventilatory capacity of the contralateral lung and the venous return to the heart.

Clinical Presentation/Examination

The most common presenting symptoms in a patient with pneumothorax are chest pain and shortness of breath. The pain is often pleuritic and radiates to the ipsilateral shoulder. Patients may also present with vague symptoms of anxiety, cough, and fatigue. Patients with secondary SP are more likely to be symptomatic because of the underlying lung disease. Physical examination findings become prominent as the patient develops tension physiology. Typical signs seen in a patient with a pneumothorax include the following:

- Distant or absent breath sounds
- Tachypnea
- Asymmetric chest expansion
- Use of accessory muscles

- Tachycardia
- Hypotension
- Jugular venous distention

Diagnostic Procedures/Treatment

Management depends on a primary versus secondary cause. In primary SP, after the initial event, patients are at an approximately 30% risk of experiencing a recurrent episode.[18] Most commonly, patients are not offered surgical intervention for the first event, but a second event warrants treatment. In patients at high risk for problems related to a pneumothorax, such as airline pilots and scuba divers, intervention is typically offered with the first event.

Regardless of the cause, the treatment of a symptomatic patient involves drainage of the pleural space and reexpansion of the lung. In an asymptomatic patient with a small pneumothorax, simple observation is acceptable. Drainage can be accomplished by aspiration with an intravenous or thoracentesis catheter; however, success rates are often low.[19] Placement of a traditional chest tube or pigtail catheter is the treatment of choice for an unstable or significantly symptomatic patient. In most patients, the air leak seals once the lung is fully reexpanded, but a prolonged leak beyond 7 days is an indication for surgical intervention, provided the lung is fully inflated with the aid of additional chest tubes or pigtail catheters as necessary, often with CT guidance. The CT scans should be performed with the existing tubes on suction to evaluate for incomplete lung expansion.

Definitive surgical treatment options consist of open thoracotomy versus video-assisted thoracic surgery (VATS) technique. A transaxillary thoracotomy provides excellent exposure, and the incision is hidden in the axilla. In patients with primary pneumothorax, the source is almost always small blebs at the apex of the upper lobe or on the superior segment of the lower lobe. If blebs are present, they should be excised. After excision of any disease, an effective pleurodesis needs to be performed. This procedure is key, because the underlying goal is to prevent the lung from collapsing when new blebs occur in the future. This goal is more readily accomplished with the open technique, which has led to lower recurrence rates with an open versus VATS approach. The gold standard approach with a rate of recurrence of less than 1% is an open approach with resection of blebs and pleurectomy/pleurodesis.[15] However, this rate of recurrence must be weighed against the increased patient discomfort associated with this procedure. A VATS approach may be less uncomfortable but seems to have a recurrence rate as high as 5%.[20]

Summary

Spontaneous pneumothorax can be either primary or secondary in nature. All symptomatic patients should be managed with drainage. The decision to surgically treat for prevention of recurrence depends on the cause and, to some extent, the risk associated with recurrence. VATS is a less morbid procedure; however, it has an increased risk of failure.

PULMONARY EMPYEMA
Introduction

Pulmonary empyema is the collection of suppurative fluid in the pleural space (**Fig. 2**). This condition can be from a thoracic injury, secondary to an underlying pneumonia, or a parapneumonic effusion. The American Thoracic Society breaks an empyema down in to 3 stages: early exudative, intermediate fibrinopurulent, and late organizing.[21]

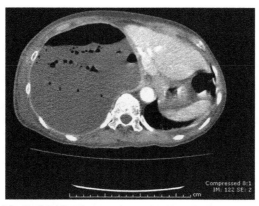

Fig. 2. Empyema with air fluid level.

Historically, drainage of an empyema was performed with an open technique, with an associated 70% mortality.[22] The advent of closed tube drainage significantly improved this mortality.

Clinical Presentation/Examination

A high index of suspicion is needed to make the diagnosis of empyema. Patients typically present with subtle symptoms, most commonly failure to thrive, with anorexia, weight loss, and poor energy. Symptoms, including fever, cough, tachypnea, desaturation, and leukocytosis are usually associated with the underlying cause, such as pneumonia, and are not always present. A common cause of empyema is infection of a pleural effusion in the setting of pneumonia.

Diagnosis

When a chest radiograph or CT scan shows a pleural fluid collection, fluid sampling and analysis are the first steps in deciding the appropriate treatment. If the effusion is loculated, air fluid levels may be apparent on plain film. The diagnosis of empyema is based on the composition of the fluid and the radiographic characteristics. The fluid has different characteristics based on the stage of the empyema (**Table 1**). These findings are determined by imaging and examination of the fluid. Although an organizing peel defines the late stage, CT and ultrasonography are not uniformly predictive for diagnosis.

Table 1
Stages of pulmonary empyema

	Early	Intermediate	Late
Fluid characteristics (≥1 of the following)	pH <7.2 Glucose <40 mg/dL Lactate dehydrogenase >1000 IU/dL Protein >2.5 g/dL White blood cell count >500/μL Specific gravity >1.018	Thick opaque fluid Positive culture	Organizing peel with entrapment of the lung

Management

Once the diagnosis of empyema has been made, attention to removal of the purulent fluid and reexpansion of the lung are critical. If an empyema is in the early stage, a thoracentesis and antibiotics may be adequate treatment. The antibiotics are not initiated for treatment of the empyema but for treatment of the underlying pneumonia. In the absence of an underlying pneumonia, no antibiotics should be used, because they cannot enter the pleural space and therefore offer no benefit to the patient. For patients with an underlying pneumonia, empirical antibiotics should be started while awaiting culture results of the fluid based on the common causes of infection. For community-acquired pneumonia with empyema, streptococcal and anaerobic infections are most common and multidrug-resistant *Staphylococcus* is most commonly found in hospital-acquired pneumonia with empyema.[23]

For larger single homogeneous fluid collections, drainage with a chest tube is recommended. The size of the chest tube was initially believed to be important. However, recent studies have shown that smaller-bore chest tubes have similar outcomes to larger chest tubes. After drainage, a CT scan should be obtained to look for residual fluid. Streptokinase or another form of lytic therapy can be used to decrease the need for operative intervention; however, the data on outcomes are mixed.[24] The first-line treatment at our facility is typically 3 to 5 days of lytic therapy. After this treatment, repeat imaging should be obtained. If progress is being made, then lytic treatment should be continued. If there is no progress after 5 days, then an alternative treatment plan should be made.

The role of surgery in empyema may be declining. In the MIST1 (Multicenter Intrapleural Sepsis 1) trial,[25] only 18% of patients failed treatment with antibiotics and chest tube drainage and required operation. Patients may require VATS if there is incomplete drainage despite adequate chest tube placement and streptokinase therapy. However, in the presence of a thick peel, an open approach may be necessary.

For a persistent cavity, treatment to obliterate the space is required. The options are decortication, an Eloesser flap, thoracoplasty, or filling in the space with muscle. Determination of which approach to use depends on patient age, comorbidities, the size of the cavity, and the underlying condition of the lung.

Summary

Initial treatment of pulmonary empyema requires drainage and antibiotics. With complex and multiloculated effusions, surgical intervention may be required. An attempt at chest tube drainage with the addition of intrapleural streptokinase may obviate surgical intervention; however, results are mixed.

REFERENCES

1. Choking. Available at: http://www.nsc.org/safety_home/HomeandRecreational Safety/Pages/Choking.aspx#older%20adults. Accessed June 20, 2013.
2. McCaffrey TV. Classification of laryngotracheal stenosis. Laryngoscope 1992; 102:1335–40.
3. Yang K. Tracheal stenosis after a brief intubation. Anesth Analg 1995;80:625–7.
4. Shigemura N, Wan IY, Yu SC, et al. Multidisciplinary management of life-threatening massive hemoptysis: a 10-year experience. Ann Thorac Surg 2009; 87(3):849–53.
5. Dweik RA, Stoller JK. Role of bronchoscopy in massive hemoptysis. Clin Chest Med 1999;20(1):89–105.

6. Corey R, Hla KM. Major and massive hemoptysis: reassessment of conservative management. Am J Med Sci 1987;294(5):301–9.
7. Crocco JA, Rooney JJ, Tankushen DS, et al. Massive hemoptysis. Arch Intern Med 1968;121(6):495–8.
8. Hirshberg B, Biran I, Glazer M, et al. Hemoptysis: etiology, evaluation, and outcome in a tertiary referral hospital. Chest 1997;112(2):440–4.
9. Sakr L, Dutau H. Massive hemoptysis: an update on the role of bronchoscopy in diagnosis and management. Respiration 2010;80:38–58.
10. Flume PA, Yankaskas JR, Ebeling M, et al. Massive hemoptysis in cystic fibrosis. Chest 2005;128(2):729–38.
11. Cahill BC, Ingbar DH. Massive hemoptysis, assessment and management. Clin Chest Med 1994;15:147–67.
12. Van den Heuvel MM, Els A, Koegelenberg CF. Risk factors for recurrence of hae-moptysis following bronchial artery embolization for life-threatening haemoptysis. Int J Tuberc Lung Dis 2007;11:909–14.
13. Wong LT, Lillquist YP, Culham G, et al. Treatment of recurrent hemoptysis in a child with cystic fibrosis by repeated bronchial artery embolizations and long-term tranexamic acid. Pediatr Pulmonol 1996;22:275–9.
14. Jean-Baptise E. Clinical assessment and management of massive hemoptysis. Crit Care Med 2000;28:1642–7.
15. MacDuff A, Arnold A, Harvey J. Management of spontaneous pneumothorax: British Thoracic Society Pleural Disease Guideline 2010. Thorax 2010;65(Suppl 2):ii18–31.
16. Bense L, Eklund G, Wiman LG. Smoking and the increased risk of contracting spontaneous pneumothorax. Chest 1987;92:1009–12.
17. Grundy S, Bentley A, Tschopp JM. Primary spontaneous pneumothorax: a diffuse disease of the pleura. Respiration 2012;83:185–9.
18. Gobbel W. Spontaneous pneumothorax. J Thorac Cardiovasc Surg 1963;46:331–45.
19. Baumann MH, Strange C. Treatment of spontaneous pneumothorax: a more aggressive approach? Chest 1997;112:789–804.
20. Hatz RA, Kaps MF, Meimarakis G, et al. Long-term results after video-assisted thoracoscopic surgery for first-time and recurrent spontaneous pneumothorax. Ann Thorac Surg 2000;70:253–7.
21. Andrews NC, Parker EF, Shaw RP, et al. Management of nontuberculous empyema. Am Rev Respir Dis 1962;85:935–6.
22. Peters RM. Empyema thoracis: historical perspective. Ann Thorac Surg 1989;48:306–8.
23. Maskell NA, Batt S, Hedley EL, et al. The bacteriology of pleural infection by genetic and standard methods and its mortality significance. Am J Respir Crit Care Med 2006;174:817–23.
24. Cameron R, Davies HR. Intra-pleural fibrinolytic therapy versus conservative management in the treatment of adult parapneumonic effusions and empyema. Cochrane Database Syst Rev 2008;(2):CD002312.
25. Maskell NA, Davies CW, Nunn AJ, et al. Controlled trial of intrapleural streptoki-nase for pleural infection. N Engl J Med 2005;352:865–74.

Index

Note: Page numbers of article titles are in **boldface** type.

A

Abdomen
    open, **131–153**. *See also* Open abdomen; Open-abdomen technique
Abdominal compartment syndrome (ACS), 132–135
    classification of, 132–133
    diagnosis of, 134
    introduction, 132
    management of, 134–135
    pathophysiology of, 133–134
    prevalence of, 133
    risk factors for, 134
Abdominal wall
    anterior
        anatomy of, 102–103
Abdominal wall closure
    temporary, 137–144
Acalculous cholecystitis, 7
ACS. *See* Abdominal compartment syndrome (ACS)
Acute cholangitis, 8
Acute cholecystitis
    calculous, 5–7
Acute inflammatory surgical diseases, **1–30**. *See also specific diseases, e.g.,* Appendicitis
    acute cholecystitis/cholangitis, 5–8
    acute pancreatitis, 9–15
    Clostridium difficile colitis, 20–25
    diverticulitis, 15–20
    introduction, 1–2
Acute mesenteric ischemia, **165–181**
    anatomy and physiology related to, 166–169
    clinical presentation of, 171–172
    diagnosis of, 171–172
    diseases leading to, 165–166
    management of, 172–175
    outcome of, 179
    overview, 165–166
    pathophysiology of, 169–171
Acute obstruction, **77–96**
    biliary, 90–91
    colonic, 86–90
    described, 77

Surg Clin N Am 94 (2014) 193–202
http://dx.doi.org/10.1016/S0039-6109(13)00183-7
0039-6109/14/$ – see front matter © 2014 Elsevier Inc. All rights reserved.

surgical.theclinics.com

Moving?

Make sure your subscription moves with you!

To notify us of your new address, find your **Clinics Account Number** (located on your mailing label above your name), and contact customer service at:

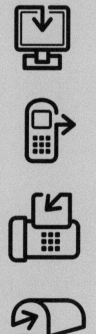

Email: journalscustomerservice-usa@elsevier.com

800-654-2452 (subscribers in the U.S. & Canada)
314-447-8871 (subscribers outside of the U.S. & Canada)

Fax number: 314-447-8029

Elsevier Health Sciences Division
Subscription Customer Service
3251 Riverport Lane
Maryland Heights, MO 63043

*To ensure uninterrupted delivery of your subscription, please notify us at least 4 weeks in advance of move.

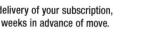

Printed and bound by CPI Group (UK) Ltd, Croydon, CR0 4YY

12/10/2024

01773480-0001